C000173886

Finally Climbing My Tree

Lost 70lbs
Found Myself

JEREMY DAVIS

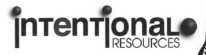

intentional
RESOURCES

Published by **intentional resources limited**

Copyright © 2012 by Jeremy Davis

First Published 2012

ISBN 978-0-9574359-0-2

Printed in England by Tyson Colour

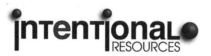

admin@intentionalgroup.co.uk

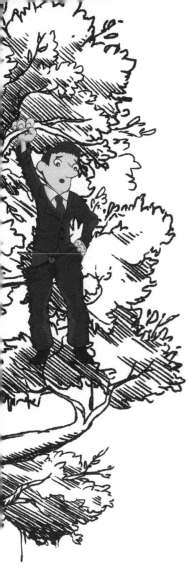

Contents

Appendices

» Sample Menus and Meals
» Links to Useful Material

Acknowledgments

There are so many people I need to thank who have played a part in my weight loss journey, from helping me discover how I could lose weight, to motivating me to lose the pounds and finally by encouraging me to write this book.

To **Hayley** and **Claire**, you had no idea that what you did inspired me to start and made me dream it could happen!

John at Powerhouse Fitness and **Nick** at Evolution Slimming, thanks for listening to me and helping me find the right equipment to start me on the road to success

To **Sjoerd**, I will miss you but your influence will never be forgotten.

Friends like **Cathy**, **Vicki**, **Jonathan** and **Jooles**, your desire to help me get this project fully completed inspired me so much to crack on. You are amazing.

Thanks **to all my buddies** for their kind words, warm hearts and amazing support, for helping me believe and then caring enough to ask how I managed it.

Finally to my darling wife **Lisa** who shows me her beauty inside and out every day of our lives together.

Preface

Finally Climbing My Tree is the story of Jeremy Davis, who over an 8-month period dropped 70 pounds. This dramatic weight loss has been somewhat noticeable, and many people have asked for the secret of Jeremy's success as they too search for an answer to one of their own big challenges in life – how to lose unwanted weight and keep it off. It is a personal tale of why Jeremy went on this life changing journey and how he achieved his weight loss.

This book is not about diets but all about facing challenges and intentionally taking steps that keep the reader focused on their personal motivations and behaviours to give each person the best possible opportunity to achieve their own weight goals. It asks many questions which readers are encouraged to answer honestly, as well as tips on what worked for Jeremy and what did not! It's all aimed at making the weight loss challenge less complex and easier to understand.

Jeremy invites you to join him on an exciting, heartfelt and sometimes crazy journey to see what might possibly be waiting for you if or when you INTENTIONALLY take control of your life!

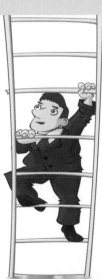

Introduction

I have never considered myself a writer, however here I am writing down my experiences of the last year - but only after having had so many people ask me to write about how I managed to do it! The "it" to which I refer is how I finally lost 70lbs in weight and permanently changed my life!

To answer the question of "how I did it" will take a little while but over the course of this book I'll share my experiences and hopefully encourage you to be able to do the same. If I can do it, you certainly can.

Who am I to write a 'diet book'?
So what are my qualifications for undertaking this task? I hear you shouting out already! First I should tell you a little about myself. I am married to Lisa, we have two wonderful children Joshua and Laura who are 13 and 11 but seem to think they are 27 and 19. I am in many ways an average guy with a job, a house and a car. However, I have also battled with my weight for many years but finally I have managed to lose the excess flab and I've kept it off.

I've always been of the opinion that if you want to try something new or have some help with a difficult activity then it's best to ask someone who can actually do it or who has proved they're capable! If I wanted to learn to put up shelves I would ask someone who has significant DIY experience, someone who has put shelves up on the wall that are level and have stayed there for a while. If I wanted to learn how to start a business, I would make a beeline for someone who had started their own!

In the British TV comedy programme 'Little Britain' one sketch makes me roar with laughter – it features a weight loss coach who is distinctly chubby. The whole premise of the sketch is that she cannot control her own weight let alone anyone else's, and her catch phrase of "we all love a bit of cake!" sums up so well her attitude to the whole subject of weight loss. We laugh because we know deep down that this is not a good advert for success.

So, my major qualification, as I embark on writing this book, is that I am able to stand before you as someone who has walked the very road you are travelling right now. I am not talking from theory. I am not commenting having merely watched other people lose weight. I am simply someone who knew that they needed to get thinner yet just could not seem to do it but who, after lots of research worked out a way to succeed.

In my professional career I am a Global Project Manager and my roles have all had a common theme, namely making the complex seem simpler! So after years of fighting the scales, it finally dawned on me that I needed to manage my weight loss in exactly the same way.

Undoubtedly, the whole subject of weight loss has been complicated by certain parts of an industry that has specialised in making the simple seem complex. Very soon I discovered that, contrary to what I'd spent a lifetime believing, losing weight didn't have to be complicated or daunting.

My previous life of fear

So here I am, a person who has lived through most of the fears you can imagine about weight loss.

How to start, what to do, when to do it? Am I allowed to ever eat again? Will my life from now on be a miserable existence where I am only allowed to eat one carrot every other day? Am I disciplined enough to cope, or will I feel like a failure when I 'relapse' and eat something that is not so healthy? Will I feel guilty yet again?

The prospect of losing weight comes with hundreds of questions just like these and like most dieters I think I altered my worries on a daily basis.   Variety is the spice of life! In truth, I spent most of my life scared of some form of failure when it came to my weight. Does this sound familiar?

Once I had done a whole heap of thinking, which I will explain in detail, I started my journey.I was not looking for a miracle cure, nor did I find one. I certainly did not want to reinvent the dieting wheel, but I was convinced that the right course of action did exist for me. I just needed to keep it simple and work to a plan. *In many of the later chapters, you will find me writing about being "Intentional" and I commend this word to you right now as we start together. I wanted to do things deliberately by choice, not because I could not help myself.*

Please understand I am trying to explain what worked for me. *In truth, dieting is simple - just eat less and exercise more!* However, as those of us who battle with our weight know, there's some really complex misinformation out there which makes our lives very tricky.   I do not in any way encourage you to do as I did, but I want to give you the chance to see the road map that kept me safe. By sharing my experiences, I want to help you to stimulate your own thinking.

This book and lifestyle is based on one simple premise. *I truly do believe that the whole ethos of a "diet" is flawed.*

To my mind, diets do not seem to work very well or at least very often. Many eating schemes, of course, do work for losing some pounds but the real issue is making weight loss stick and keeping to that lower weight for the long term.

Sections of the diet industry seem to spend a significant amount of time encouraging people to try the latest diet fashion and when that does not work to stem the tide of obesity within our world it just invents a new theory. I speak as someone who has ridden the merry-go-round that is the diet industry. There are no new theories or fads left for me and now I have decided to get off and do something different, which works for me. I have chosen to be very honest and speak openly about the various dieting activities which I have lived through and to comment on my experiences. Some are very positive indeed, some less so, and I will happily acknowledge when and where I have received positive assistance from a regime or part of it .

Also, I cannot and will not pretend that all dieters have the same issues or that my way of seeing things is the only valid view of this particular subject. What I will say however, is that I wish that when I started to lose weight 25 years ago I had known the simple facts, which I will explain as we journey through this book together. I will also reveal many of the questions I asked myself and I will also share the answers I discovered.

If I had known at the start what I know now, I am convinced I would have got to my final destination much faster and with far less pain.

So what is this weight loss programme about?
I could provide you with hundreds of graphs and charts, which would prove we have a weight problem in our society and yet I have chosen not to do so. You see, I know that during all my years of struggle, when I was trying to get thinner, deep inside *I knew I had to lose weight. Not society, but me!* I figure that if you have read this far, you may have come to the same conclusion. So let's not worry about society, let's just worry about you and see if we can use my experiences to make your personal weight loss journey easier, quicker and less painful.

This book is a personal programme that will do everything it can to help you focus on your lifestyle rather than focusing on a prescribed diet of "eat this, eat that and stand on one leg while you do it!"

The very idea of forcing someone to give up a whole food group and then wondering how on earth they live a fulfilled life seems bonkers to me.

If you had told me at any point in the past 25 years that I could lose 70lbs in just eight months, and keep the weight off, I would never have believed you. I know so many people who, like me, have 'yoyo-ed' up and down with their weight and I believe it all comes down to one simple problem. The moment we have lost the pounds, we have reverted to the same behaviours and eating patterns that got us to the size we were when we began dieting. On each attempt we've become more disheartened as we added another failure to our personal list of failed diet attempts. Shall I give you all the facts and figures and percentages involved in global 'failed dieting'? No, I won't do that now or at any point in the book.

This book is not about the problems that others face, this is personal - just between me and you. Before we go any further, there is one point to clarify:
The difficult subject of taking Medication and knowing you can still lose weight.
As with all weight loss programmes, it's about YOU working out what is safe for YOU. All diets recommend you speak to your doctor to ensure that your particular circumstances are managed in a safe way. This book is no different, and you MUST speak to your doctor about how to manage your medication while losing pounds. In my situation, of course, it was different. You see I was on three different medications, each of which had a side effect of weight increase. This meant that I had told myself I was so large as a direct result of my medication and not as a result of eating too much, or my general lifestyle. I truly empathise with anyone with similar challenges and know that making sure a diet does not interfere with your medication is vital. As you will read later, though, my medication was a great excuse and fed into my "victim" status when it came to my weight. So whilst I cannot draw any direct link with your circumstances, I can clearly say I was wrong, and I managed to find a way to manage my medications and my weight loss.

Eight years ago I was rushed to hospital with ridiculously high blood pressure and as a result I have to take a pill that slows my heart rate. For me, it was vital I understood that I needed advice on how to exercise safely.

All of the people YOU may need to talk to should be very obvious. People who are overweight will be told by their doctor, on just about every visit that they need to lose weight or would benefit from being lighter. The fact that you are reading this introduction means you have started on an exciting road but please take talking to people very seriously. Please speak to friends, family, experts, doctors or whoever can help you!

I was sad that I was so large. I was scared that I would fail, and everything inside me made me want to do this silently without speaking to anyone about it. I am delighted I fought that urge and spoke to experts - people who had done what I wanted to do or people who knew their stuff!

This book is my journey. It is the story of my road to success, not through some new fad diet, nor with a cure-all magic pill. This book is written simply with a heart to take you through my experience, to explain what went well and what went not so well, my hopes, my fears and how I in the end managed to both lose the weight and keep it off!

Life is fun when you share
There is no doubt I could not have managed to have finally achieved my weight loss without the support of my gorgeous wife, Lisa. She has always been wonderful in having and loving a larger-sized husband. When I needed to begin this process, as you will hear in the book, she did not tell me I needed to drop the pounds but she simply came with me! Thank you my love.

The failure of being heavy – my confession
I will never forget the day that I finally knew something had to change. It is a true story and one that will always stick in my head.

I love Center Parcs – the holiday parks for families that are found in the UK and Europe. My family love spending vacations there and we have been blessed to go many times.   Lisa is brilliant at organising these trips and always makes sure we have booked activities well in advance to make the best of our time there.
She is so talented and great at keeping us organised that we have named her "Tour Guide Tilly".

A few years ago Center Parcs started to install some wonderful tree-rope-type adventures, and the pictures in the brochure seemed amazing. Josh and Laura were so excited, and we were just about to book a trip into the treetops when we spotted the bad news. "Maximum Weight: 15st".

Now, at this point, I was 17st 11lbs with just 10 weeks to go before we arrived at the centre in Elveden, Norfolk in Eastern England. Short of cutting off my leg, I was never going to get down to that weight before the holiday. I insisted Lisa took the kids into the trees. Inside I was destroyed. The pain I felt at not being about to undertake this part of our holiday is really hard to describe. I felt I had let Lisa down, had let the kids down and was a disappointment to all of them. None of that is true and, of course, I was not a disappointment to anyone but that is genuinely how I felt. Watching them laugh and giggle as they climbed was such a mixed feeling. I was thrilled my family enjoyed the trees yet so upset *I was not making memories with them but watching them make memories without me.*

Those who know the Elveden Center Parcs will know that there is also a boating lake. We decided we would spend some time together on the water. When we got there we discovered what I can only describe as an inflatable giant hamster wheel that floated on the water. The kids were so excited, but yet again I was too heavy to participate. For a second time, I had to say "no". My kids were super about not spinning on the water but I was really struggling.

To make amends, we all decided to go out on a boat and enjoy rowing on the water but as a safety precaution everyone had to wear a life jacket. I went for the XL size and therefore the largest life jacket and with a significant amount of breathing in I managed to get the blessed thing to do up! At least something just about fitted.

That holiday, I determined that as soon as I could, I was going to go back to Center Parcs and would climb those trees and ropes, with Lisa and my family. Isn't it strange the things that upset us and the things that motivate us? I wonder if you have had similar things or times in your life that have caused you sadness?

If you do, please read on and you may find some of the answers you need to remove that upset once and for all. Certainly you will discover why the book is called *Finally Climbing My Tree!*

You have nothing to lose - but your fears, your failures and a whole lot of weight.
Please do read to the end of this book. If once you get there you think, "Nah! That's not for me" I will not be offended. If you or just one other person thinks "if Jez can do

it, so can I" then the whole process of writing it all down will have been worthwhile for me.

However, I cannot leave this introduction without telling you I DID return to Center Parcs with some good friends. I DID climb those trees with my wife and children, I DID, in fact, do everything I wanted to do and the folks at Center Parcs made me feel wonderful when I told them my story.

If you have had similar experiences, please read on, and also learn how to make a whole new series of memories.

Chapter One
Motivation

Getting thinner has been a dream of mine for so many years. I cannot remember the number of times I have tried to do it. I also cannot remember the number of times I have bought into the next diet - some sensible, and some not so sensible! I have not gone back and counted the number of attempts, but it is fair to say that diets and me have not been a raging success.

I have focused on carbohydrates, on proteins, on shakes, on missing meals. I've failed at each attempt and like many people I have found that every time I have finished dieting I am in fact heavier than when I started! Now, I'm not mad, at least that's what I thought, but I am sure the basic idea of this activity is to weigh less at the end and not more! Of course, every time I failed, it reinforced one fact - I was not in control of my food destiny.

These constant failures made the activity of truly getting healthy harder in two ways. Firstly, I felt even more of a failure. Another dieting fiasco. Just who was I kidding? I processed the situation like this - "dieting has failed for me, but the diet works, it has to work because there is a whole industry telling me it works, so it must be ME and my hopelessness that has stopped this diet working".

My thought processes were subtle, but that was the message none the less.

Secondly, of course, I now found myself a few pounds heavier than when I last started dieting. Unless I had grown a few inches in height, to keep my Body Mass Index (BMI) in equilibrium I now not only had my original weight to lose but also a few more pounds, so the journey just got longer.

The power of other success stories!
So what made me change my thinking and set me off on the right way forward? As ever, it was several things that happened around the same time to point me in a certain direction.

Lisa and I had reason to visit some friends in Southampton, on the south coast of

England, and when we arrived we were introduced to a lovely lady called Hayley.

Hayley looks like a typically healthy woman. I'm sure, nothing more than a dress size 10. However, as the conversation proceeded I discovered this amazing looking woman had lost 9 stone in weight in a single year. Yes that's right - 126lbs! As it transpired she went on to win Slimming World's "Regional Slimmer of the Year" Award and I believe she was second overall in the United Kingdom in 2012. Simply amazing!

Hayley and I had not met before and the fact she had lost so much weight was a real challenge to me. Why Hayley and not me?

At this point, I want to focus on two aspects of my meeting with Hayley. Firstly, when I saw Hayley I saw a smart, bright, confident young mother. It did not even enter my head that she had ever been 'large'. I had not known Hayley before she was her current slim size, and she was in such great shape that you really would never know she had dieted. Right in front of me there was evidence of what a 'fresh start' looked like. It slowly began to dawn on me that if I could finally sort out this weight business, there was a world for me where people would view me in a new way rather than just as Jez, that nice, happy, large chap.

Secondly, she was passionate about her weight loss. Not boring, just passionate. Hayley and I sat, we talked and I don't think she knew what she had started within me. She was helping and did not even know it. I love this type of help. Inspire and then be supportive of other people. Always have an eye on what you can give, and not what you can receive.

You'll recall that Hayley used Slimming World to lose her excess weight, and it obviously worked for her. I do think women can sometimes find belonging to clubs a great source of strength and support. Hayley has now established a Slimming World group and if ever you want to see another example of someone who is not telling others what to do but simply sharing her passion for helping others lose weight, then Hayley is your woman!

Yet I knew that I could never win the weight loss war with that type of system. I had failed twice before with the 'weight club' approach but that was a commentary on me not the system. As I've said, there are many ways to lose weight and I'm not about to tell you which route to take, but instead this book is designed to deal with the process of succeeding, mastering your fears and finding that new lifestyle which will keep you in the best shape for the rest of your life.

Then there was Claire. She is a dear friend and has a totally different story. She attends the local Salvation Army church where we are both members. She lost 4 stones (56lbs) and looks amazing. I saw her lose the weight week by week and it was just a fantastic achievement. I was so proud of her, and simply marvelled at the self-control she seemed to have discovered. Once again, in the nicest possible way, I wondered "Why Claire and not me?"

Well of course the truth was that Claire had decided that she was going to take action. She was not going to moan and whine that she had SO much weight to lose. She was not going to sit on her backside and ignore her feelings. She started to eat more healthily and began to exercise. She achieved a wonderful result in a totally different way to Hayley, yet was equally as successful.

Let's not forget the most important issue in this weight loss game. It's not to lose the most weight but to have a healthy lifestyle and a healthy BMI. Although once I also decided to take control of my life and my weight and I lost 70lbs, I could never have lost as much as Hayley, because then I would have been unhealthy. I would have been painfully thin if I had lost 9 stones. No, each of us takes a unique journey and we need to understand what WE each need to do, for ourselves.

After considering these two very special ladies and their wonderful achievements, I started to think more broadly about the people I knew who had lost weight. The more I thought about it, the more I realised that the vast majority of the folks I knew who had lost a significant amount of weight were women. Why was it that men seemed so less able to lose significant amounts of weight? Was it the motivation? Was it all in the genes? Or was it that women cared more about their own health and their appearance? Who knows?

The damage was done. My Center Parcs nightmare was in my head, the girls had proved it could be done and that was that, I was ready to start the most exciting self-discovery journey of my life.

After talking to my female friends, I had the distinct impression they enjoyed, or were at the very least comfortable, imparting a few really simple basic truths about WHY they had lost the weight.

They wanted to look good. I am sure that in a professional 'diet book' I am supposed to write that their main motivation was healthy lifestyle but this book is meant to be real, I want you to understand what we truly feel, not what others think we should feel. Secondly, the dieters with kids were keen to set a better example to their children. They also wanted to feel more energetic, and finally, they wished to live a longer life.

Why is it that so many men have such a problem admitting that they want to look good, or feel good? It seems to me there are two definite camps. There are the guys who do not care how they look or who do not care enough to do something positive about it. I counted myself a fine example of this group. My personal excuses went as follows – 'there are lots of reasons why I'm too large, lots of medication, travel lots for work, and lots of eating out for work.' I am sure you can fill in the rest but in truth I had just not been bothered enough to do anything about my weight.

The other group of people is found at the opposite end of the spectrum and seems to be obsessed with fitness. They are found at the gym every two minutes, getting fitter and stronger and are normally all muscle. Well, I certainly did not fancy that!

I am just a normal guy. I wanted to be fitter and healthier than I was, and I wanted to feel more attractive to my wife. I did want to feel that I looked good, and was prepared to put the effort in to achieve it. But did I want to spend every spare moment in the gym?

I am also a proud Dad, proud of our kids and all they are. Yet I am also a proud Dad in another way and I figure they deserve to have me around for a long time, to be able to spend quality time with them and play with them, unimpeded by Health and Safety rules. I was certainly committed to that and was about to make it happen.

At work, I often use a phrase that goes like this:
"I can't hear the words you are saying as your actions are speaking so loudly"

I have no idea where I first heard it and I apologise if I have quoted someone without credit. However, I do know that it is true. I needed to stop thinking words or feeling words and let my actions start to speak.

Decision Time
It was time for me to ask myself some tough questions.

Ever since I was at school I have carried a little too much weight. In fact, I cannot remember a time when I was not aware of being overweight. When it came to sports, and 'PE' I dreaded cross country in particular. Endurance sports were so hard for me to complete. I did enjoy racket sports like tennis and badminton and as for running I was deadly over 3 metres!

I was very self-aware through my youth and twenties, far more so really than my size dictated, but when I was larger I found it did not matter what positive messages I received, I only focused on the negatives. This proved to me that I was a victim of my weight. It was time for me to decide on my future.

You will find that some of the chapters in this book end with a series of questions aimed at allowing you to see what I was doing but also to give you a framework for what you can do in YOUR circumstances.

Here are some of the questions I asked myself at the time I made the decision to start taking my weight loss seriously:

1. Having heard the stories from my friends who had managed to reach their weight goals, did I think I could truly do the same?
2. As I had struggled in the past, was I prepared to start approaching weight loss in a different way?
3. Different actions were needed to get different results so was I now ready to stop the talking and actually do something different?
4. Was I a victim of my circumstances or were the excuses I had come up with over the years just convenient whitewash?
5. Was there anything out of my control that might stop me either starting or completing this adventure?
6. If the answer to number 5 was nothing, was I now prepared to take the first step to deliver on my deep, long term desire to be the best "me" I could be?

Once I had answered these questions honestly, I was fully committed. I knew that if any issue at all was within my control nothing was going to stop me.

I was aware that there were some challenges that I would need to meet head-on, like the amount of time I spent working overseas and entertaining, but I was now up for doing something different and this time I was determined that I would achieve different results.

Chapter Two
Vision...The New Me and the Benefits

How confusing is this?
As I embarked on this new and determined weight loss journey, the first thing I decided I needed was information. So I headed for the internet.

Oh my goodness, how many websites are dedicated to dieting?!?!

I was utterly amazed – there are literally hundreds and hundreds of diet websites. To prove my point, try this little game. I want you to try to create a new diet title. Use three words. The first must be "The" and the last must be the word "Diet". You can insert any and every word that even vaguely makes sense to you and be assured you will find a diet identified by the middle word in your fantastic new diet regime.

I tried the game and got bored after 75 attempts. 'The From Fat to Thin Diet ', 'The First to Last Diet' and 'The range of emotions including Happiness, Pleasure, Bliss, Lifestyle and on and on Diet'. The food and exercise programmes just kept coming.

By investigating so many websites I made my first discovery - I had no idea what I was doing. There were sites telling me to eat more protein, and others to eat less protein. Some were disciples of carbohydrate management, some prescribed fasting and others told me I could eat as much as I liked. There were those who emphasized extreme exercise with fat free, small meals, eating little but often. Some diet programmes were all about pills, and some were about potions, and some I truly never did understand.

However, I did notice that for every diet website that told me one thing, I could find another that told me near as the exact opposite. I could feel the old sense of panic setting in again as I searched aimlessly for the best way to diet. Here I was, a guy used to running projects worth millions of pounds and still this world was baffling.

Is this for a few months or for life?
While I was researching what felt like every diet in the universe, in several places I read that diets did not work. This seemed a little strange but bearing in mind

everything else I had read was proving to be utterly contradictory, it started to make sense.

I decided to think about this for a while. At school I was taught about 'cause and effect' - every action has an equal and opposite reaction. I could not remember the detail but I could recall that this meant that if you hit a snooker ball into a stationary snooker ball it moved!

I decided to undertake some research at my local diner. Here they sold all types of food. Salads, burgers, chips, jacket potatoes, vegetarian food, chicken, beef, you get the picture, it's a very a wide menu. I noticed one particular trend. Not all, but in the majority of cases, the people who were overweight were tucking into large plates of food and the people who appeared smaller tended to have smaller plates of food in front of them.

Then I asked myself "I wonder who is on a diet?" It was about a second after this thought hit, that I FINALLY had my "eureka" moment. *I had no idea who was on a diet and it really didn't matter. If I ate 2,500 calories a day from that moment on, I would become a thinner person. What had been eaten in the past was totally and utterly irrelevant. I had discovered that the past was gone and I could only control what I ate from that moment on. I was at the point of a new beginning.*

There it was and it was so simple and right before my eyes. I could use any diet if it helped me lose weight quickly but I knew that I would simply return to my old self plus a few pounds once I left the diet plan and began eating in the old way!

What had started out as very confusing was now so simple! Goodness I was annoyed. Why, before that momentous day, had no one ever told me this vital nugget of information?

Knowledge is indeed power and now I had the power to go forward!

Do I have other skills learned in other areas of my life that I can use for weight loss? I have been fortunate to work in some wonderful companies who have spent so much money sending me on training courses. One of the key skills of leadership is the ability to build a clear vision for people to work towards. I work for a large multi-national organisation and I've learned that *the difference that a clear vision makes to any project is simply staggering.*

8

I decided that I needed a weight loss programme that enabled me to use some of my work skills to help me drop the pounds. Easier said than done because I now needed a vision that I could own - not something abstract but something of me! What was I going to look like when I lost all the weight? Could I see a picture of what a thin Jeremy would look like? My brother, Greg, has always managed to keep on top of his weight and so I assumed I might look a little like him and it turns out I was not too far from correct. Even so, as I searched for my vision I found this to be a difficult task, and yet it did give me a strong sense of why I wanted to start this exciting journey and where it may be heading and although I struggled, I certainly began to see in my head the type of person I wanted to be.

The 'new me' was very confident and pleased with his appearance, delighted he could undertake all the activities he wished to do with his lovely family. I had a boss who assured me that I would be physically less tired with my global travel if I lost some of my weight. So in my mind I imagined that work would be easier and less stressful. I could sense the areas of change I wanted in my physical appearance and I think I got close enough to what I was trying to achieve.

I genuinely hope you can do a better job than I initially did, of seeing that picture of a thinner you in your imagination. It can be done and I know others who have managed it, it was just me that couldn't really see that clear vision at first.

As I've explained, I'm a project manager, so I also looked forward to the 'new me' in typically organized fashion. I made sure I wrote down all the key pieces of information and reminders that I might need for future reference. What were my motivations as I set out on the journey? What was I going to eventually look like? What was my target size? What activities would I eventually be able to enjoy that were not possible in the past? What would work feel like in this new world? There was much more on my list and then I didn't put it away but posted it where I would see it.

There were many moments in the first few weeks of my new weight loss regime when I really needed to remember these facts, so having the list of my dreams, hopes and expectations in my face certainly helped. If you follow a similar process the same will be true for you, I promise!

As you can see I had moved my head space from one of dreading giving up food, asking why I was doing this and fearing failure, to one of excitement and intentional anticipation. As I looked at my list, this was no longer the negative experience of the past, but the first steps of a really positive life changing experience! My "Thank You" to all my employers for teaching me the power of building a clear vision is heartfelt and what a massive difference it made.

So just what were the *tangible* benefits of intentionally starting a weight loss regime?

The real benefit of a clear vision is truly only seen when things start to get difficult. In a work situation, you can usually get all the stakeholders to agree about starting a particular project. Normally there is a clear reason for a piece of work and everyone is comfortable that action is necessary. However, all projects have days when things get tricky and usually these have little to no major consequence to anyone so do not affect the general level of commitment. However, imagine a world where the cost of a project rises and requires a bigger budget and as a result one of the stakeholders is unprepared to agree to take on extra investment. Now it gets a little awkward and it is at these moments when a clear and simply articulated benefits statement which has been agreed in advance by all partners, will save the poor Project Manager's life. Instead of getting side-tracked the document helps keep people focused on the real benefits and reasons for the activity or project.

I've found that the same is true in losing weight and changing your lifestyle. Things change along the way and even get reprioritised so having a clear determination about what you want for the future will keep you focused. How many people have faltered or let their diets simply wither and die as a result of a summer holiday or over Christmas and New Year celebrations? Having fun was more important, being with friends was more desirable than sticking to their strict food or exercise programme. Having defined and prioritised activities and goals for you and your family will put you in a good space when the difficult days come upon you, just as they did for me.

Every year my Father and I attend the National Brass Band Contest at The Royal Albert Hall in London. Every year my Mother makes us a picnic for the day which is a feast. When I started my weight loss programme, I called my lovely parents to make sure they did not forget that I was trying to become a smaller person and it would be helpful if there wasn't a lot of temptation around. If Mum had made a picnic big enough to "feed the five thousand" and I was sitting in a concert hall for eight hours, trust me I would have eaten it. This simple act – asking my parents to co-operate and work with me - was a great example of how I intended to manage any risks of my falling off the weight loss wagon. This was important and I needed to get all the people around me to understand I would start behaving differently compared to the Jeremy of old. So I shared the news. I was being very intentional in my thinking. Telling others helped them to help me and also made me feel that I was accountable for delivering on what I said I would do. There was to be no way back.

Do I allow my ego to help or to hinder me?

We are all driven by ego or pride to a greater or lesser degree. For me, I hate to tell others that I will deliver on something and then fail. As a Project Manager it should be in your DNA that failure is simply not an option. In my work life an understanding of what constitutes an action, an issue or a risk is a critical success factor. Actions need handling today, issues drive actions and so are equally handled in the present, however, if something might or could occur in the future then that is a risk.

I came to the conclusion that my ego was a huge risk when it came to getting lighter. I spoke to people about my quest, to help me see the whole journey as a positive experience and I was surrounded with encouragement. My need to get the support of others was partly driven by the need to control my own inner self and only use this "ego" in a positive way. I could have easily not told a soul that I was going to lose weight and let them simply observe the fact. However, this would have given me an easy opportunity to fail, no one would have been any the wiser that I was trying to reduce my waist size and there would have been no chance of my losing face. Therefore, when I chose to tell certain key people in my life that I was going to lose loads of weight, this was so they could help me and hold me to account. This was fully intentional. Do you have any areas of your pride that you can harness to help you on your journey?

Finally for this chapter, here are the some of the questions I had to ask myself right at the start of my journey:

1. What will I physically look like when I have got thinner?
2. How will I feel when I get to my target weight?
3. What tangible activities will I be able to undertake that I cannot at the current time?
4. How will my health improve when I complete the task?
5. Am I prepared to take a risk and tell my loved ones and friends that I will be getting thinner, and ask for their help? Could I expose my pride to potential danger by failing in public? Which people will I trust?
6. Do I truly dare to be different and specify in detail the ways in which I will change in the future?

7. Do I understand that the past is gone? What is important is only what I eat from today, going forward and letting go of the past. What has been devoured in the past is no longer important.
8. Have I finally got it into my head that diets are temporary and I need to make changes that will stick for good not just for a few months?
9. Can I decide to make a shortlist of the diets I would consider and make a decision on a personal pathway to weight loss now I know that the diet was not the important bit?
10. How will I change my lifestyle? Can I detail the changes, what I will start to do and what I will stop doing right now?

You might like to think about some of these questions and I hope it helps in your decisions on the best way forward for you. I spent time working out if I could think of little changes which might help me, ultimately, to lose weight, but in the end I decided I wanted to have rapid results so I determined to go for this in a big way!

Chapter Three

Ready...Steady...Go!

Now feels like the time I should tell you all about my starting weights, sizes and some of the targets that I set myself.

	ME	YOU
Age:	44	....
Gender:	Male	....
Height:	6ft 0 in	....
Starting Weight:	249lbs	....
Waist Size:	42 in	....
Chest Size:	48 in	....
Hip Size:	48 in	....
BMI:	33.80	....
Clinical definition:	Obese	....
Target Weight:	178lbs	....
Target loss:	71lbs	....

Sorry if this is all a bit geeky but if I was going to know where I wanted to be, I had to know from where I was starting, and certainly had to be really honest with myself. If you feel up to it you could fill in your own statistics in the available space, but if you want to keep reading, gain a little more courage and confidence and come back to the chart later, that's fine as well.

My target weight on the chart was calculated using one of the many excellent sites on the web that calculates Body Mass Index (BMI). On the internet you will read hundreds of articles which discuss BMI and ask whether or not it is a good indicator because for people with high muscle definition (aka body builders) it gives incorrect scores.

Well, I was not a body builder! Are you a body builder? If you are then please use a different guide, if not then *for the vast majority of the population, BMI it is a great tool.* In writing this book I wondered about explaining how it is calculated and have made a conscious decision just to recommend you use one of the many internet tools. All you need is your height and weight and one of the calculators will give you the ratio.

Put simply, BMI gives you a score:

Underweight:	Under 18
Normal Weight:	18-25
Overweight:	25-29.99
Obese:	30.39.99
Morbidly Obese:	40 plus

As you can see from my scores, I was well into the "Obese" section and not at all happy. Yet I needed to see it and to actually write down on a piece of paper the word OBESE before the reality of my situation really hit me. I'm not one to harbour hatred for anyone or anything but I hated the word OBESE.

A few years ago there was a big debate as to what word doctors should use when discussing this issue with their patients. Should they be referred to as "too fat" or "obese", "Too fat" was regarded as likely to hurt people's feelings. Well for me "obese" was far worse! It is not the word that is the problem, but that inner acknowledgment that my weight might lead to me dying earlier than I should if I did not do anything about it.

The BMI calculation website I used also decided to tell me that if 100 men of my age and height were standing in a line, placed in weight order, I would be number 92 in the queue! I was in the top 10% of heaviest men for my age and height! Yet again I fought back the pain. However, it was a number and I can measure numbers to chart improvement. As a result of this I set my target to be a BMI of 24.9, or just under the healthy area of BMI scoring. As it turned out, I went a little bit further and got down to 24.1.

Are there other ways to measure your target weight?
For the sake of completeness I do want to stress there are many ways to measure
your target weight. I used BMI as it is simple and widely available. Waist to Hip
Ratio is becoming popular and the National Health Service in the UK publishes
recommendations for men and women on waist size. Although I started with BMI,
there are other routes to determining your target weight if it makes life easier for you.
My only piece of advice here is just stay constant and focused on that target, however
you arrive at it.

To weigh or not to weigh? – THAT is the question
This question causes me to pause in the story and tackle a subject that just drives
me mad. I think I have been constant in saying I want a positive world, with positive
experiences. At no point does "obsessive" get included into the list of words I want to
define myself by. However, I have read in many diet books and on many internet sites
that people who weigh each day are obsessive. What pure and utter nonsense! That
is the politest thing I can say. I believe that numbers will keep you safe. If you have
bad numbers now you will be inspired when those numbers get better each day, each
week or each month. I read one diet programme which mocked people for weighing
each morning after having emptied their bladder! I think that's the ONLY time you
should weigh yourself because it is the only time of day you will be in a constant place
regarding water retention, which can affect your weight rather dramatically. With a
small risk of sounding like my namesake from BBC's "Top Gear" programme (Mr. Jeremy
Clarkson) all I can say is "For Goodness Sake!"

If I was driving down the road and I decided that knowing my speed was optional, I
wonder what the policeman would say if, when stopped, I said to him or her,
*"Excuse me officer, I know we have a gadget that would tell me the exact speed I was
driving at, but it is obsessive to keep looking at it, so if you please I won't bother! I drive
this car every day and TRUST me I know I was only doing 38mph. So, please, go away
and forget your silly accusation that I was actually travelling at 48 miles per hour. I think
you'll find I am right, not you".*

Or we could go to the petrol station and attempt estimating the amount of petrol we
took and then wonder if we were right as we ran out of fuel in the middle lane of the
motorway!

Forgive me, but it makes me so angry that responsible people give such crass advice.
My suggestion is that you measure your weight each day or every other day, to ensure

that what you are doing is working. If you are getting heavier each day and the trend goes on for a few days, you are probably eating too much and need to look at what is causing the problem. If you don't check on yourself you will be simply blind to the facts and just guessing. Rant now officially over!

Can I *really* do this?

Where was I? Oh yes I was telling you how I was number 92 in the queue of 100 men and therefore in the top 10% of heaviest men for my age and height! Now, the most weight I had ever lost in the past was 20lbs. A self-imposed target of 71lbs nearly knocked me off course. I simply could not do it. I told myself over and over again "I can't, I truly can't do it, you will fail yet again, and you will feel worse if you do this, and you will just end up heavier!" The little voices in my head were working overtime, questioning my sanity. "Can I *really* do this?"

It was then that the reasons why I wanted to succeed and some of the motivations mentioned earlier came back to my mind. I had got through what was the hardest part so far, I had admitted to myself what was needed. I was about to start the journey and no amount of self-doubt or fear was going to stop me ***taking control of my life.***

Looking back on this pivotal moment, I now know that making this commitment and moving forward despite the fear has affected me ever since. This same commitment to taking control of my life has spread into many aspects of my life. I am not a control freak, but the things I don't do very well are now all in the firing line and I am determined to be the best Jeremy I can be.

A quick example from my domestic life is that I am now far tidier at home. Our bedroom in noticeably cleaner and I now put away many more things all over the house. Settling for second best became suboptimal in many ways! Be warned this weight loss lark can change your whole life.

Pictures of me when I started

I now have a confession to make and it's a learning point that I had on my journey and which may help you. Lots of people recommend taking pictures of yourself when you are at your heaviest. I didn't do it. I couldn't do it. Honestly, I did not want pictures of Jeremy looking so large but I now deeply regret not doing so. The motivation that can come from taking a picture every 10lbs of weight loss is huge and yet, because I was so stubborn, I did not have this source of positive energy to call on. I lived in the negative feelings I had about my body and refused to acknowledge that I needed proof of the old me.

Please remember when I talk about a positive world I mean that in every aspect of life. You are a beautiful person, but take the pictures and keep them safe. I have managed to keep one pair of trousers from that 'big Jeremy' time and on the website you will find a picture of the "new" me wearing them! I have included other general pictures on the web site at *www.finallyclimbingmytree.com*. These were of me when I weighed far more, but I do apologise for the gap that is my starting picture.

So, as I start the journey, what does a good result look like?

I wanted to end this section with this observation. A good week for me when I was on my programme was one where either:

- My weight dropped even a little
- My weight did not increase
- My waist got smaller
- My hips were thinner
- My collar size was smaller

So, to give me the best chance of getting positive news I measured my weight every day, and my three sizes (waist, hips, collar size) every week. Whenever my weight did not get lighter I was changing shape and one of my sizes was changing. I loved the positive feeling I got from KNOWING things were working and I believe that you'll get the same buzz if you try it.

Questions for you and me!

1. Have you taken all your measurements?
2. Have you calculated your BMI?
3. Do you know your ideal healthy target weight?
4. By what date do you want lose your first stone (14lbs)?
5. How long do you want to take to get to your target weight?
6. Have you written down these numbers and put them somewhere safe?

Chapter Four
My Life Saver

One of the first things I needed to help me in my new weight loss life was a clear idea of what I was eating at that moment in time. This would allow me to see what changes I needed to make to my food intake. I really do recommend taking a week to undertake this exercise. You need to make a food diary, and then work out how many calories you are eating. I went on to my iPad and downloaded an Application called "MyNetDiary". There are many different web resources so don't worry if you've not got an iPad, but I needed a system that could easily tell me exactly what I was eating. My next "Thank You" is to the team at "MyNetDiary".

This App. has been simply brilliant for me. It is quick and easy to use, it has lots of the brands of food I eat, and it remembers all of my favourites. In particular I want to focus on four really important numbers that are clearly shown on this App. and several other similar types of Application. However, forgive me for referring only to the App. I actually used.

Calories and the weighing game
For every food I ate I was able to look up the calorific content. Ninety nine times out of a hundred it was even the exact brand. Where I did not know the exact portion size I weighed everything and I was amazed when I tried to weigh out 50 grams of All Bran cereal. I was nowhere near getting it right. Remember what I said about the speedometer on the car and guessing? After some weeks of measuring you might get close to estimating a weight but I do recommend weighing everything. Make a game of it and why not involve your loved ones or friends? Measure something, anything, and see who can come closest to getting it right!

The "MyNetDiary" App. gave me a recommended number of calories which I needed to consume to hit my target weight by a specified date. The great thing is the App. will not let you go too fast. Start off at a loss of one single pound per week and see how you get on. If you think you can achieve a little more, increase to 1.5 or even 2.0lbs but not more. Using the App. is easy but if nothing else please be sure that you know how to use the calorie functions.

Fat

As well as being given a target for calories you will have a daily target number for fat intake measured in grams. My suggestion is that you do not have to follow it slavishly but use the fat target as a way of seeing what items made you go over your target weight for the day or week, and to help you identify what you could have eaten to keep you on track. Fat is important in our diet because it enables key bodily functions to work well, like ensuring our brain ticks over, so please do not cut out too much fat from your diet. Focus on calories and learn to keep fat near or near enough to the target.

Protein

Please see what I have written about fat and also look for ways of increasing your protein. It is great at helping the body repair itself and is far less calorific than carbohydrate-based foods. Learn what foods help you meet your protein target. At first, I found it really hard to take on board the recommended amount of protein, as I have a natural love of carbohydrates. But by seeing what my targets were each day and identifying how I reached them, I was able to teach myself to eat a better, healthier diet which has helped me lose the 70lbs. If you're a little confused about what proteins, carbs, fat and so on are please feel free to do a little research and at the end of the book I will also show you sample meal recipes to show you what I mean. However, make sure you understand that chicken, turkey, fish, eggs, pulses, soya and nuts all are great sources of protein and can be varied to make eating proteins a pleasure not a chore.

Carbohydrates

This area of food intake was vital for me because I simply adore carbs and I recognize that they are a high source of energy for the body. Yet research has shown that there is actually no absolute need to have carbs in a healthy diet. This is defined by our bodies being able to survive without these foods, but they would be struggling to handle anything energetic! The trouble is, we all seem to love them.

Sugars, pasta, bread, potato and cereals are all included in this food group. There are two basic types of carbohydrates - complex carbs and simple carbs and the basic difference between them is that complex carbs give out energy for longer periods of time and simple carbs give a short, high energy spike to the person eating them. It is recommended to try to eat more complex carbs than simple ones.

Complex carbs include whole grain foods like whole grain bread and cereals, oats, apricots, oranges, grapefruit, pears and plums together with salads and vegetables like broccoli, cauliflower, spinach, beans and lentils. Simple carbs are based around foods with high sugar levels. These give that energy spike and a feeling of satisfaction but increase the chances of weight gain. So anything high in sugar like sweets, beer, chocolate or jam is more risky for inducing weight gain.

This is all worth remembering as it will help you make better choices. We are supposed to get around half our calories from carbohydrates yet if I don't keep an eye on these foods my calorie intake can race away to 60 and 70% from this food group. I will always need to keep a healthy balance of carbohydrates in my diet and I can only do this by identifying and measuring what I'm eating.

MyNetDiary – a great help with numbers
As I've explained, this App. has been perfect for me. It has graphs and charts and pictures and I love it! However, most importantly it tells me how much I should be eating for my current stage of my weight loss journey.

You may have noticed I never refer to my weight loss programme as "being on a diet". This really is a key point for me because 'diets' are about giving things up. The reason we see so many people lose weight and then put it back on again is that when they reach their target weight they stop giving things up and that's when the weight piles on again and all the hard work and deprivation is wasted!

The biggest single difference between what I did to succeed and the numerous times I failed had to be...*I gave up giving things up!* This is not a diet but it is a new way of life. There is no return and no way back once you've started on this road and once you've developed this mindset! Just wait until you get to the chapter on clothing and you will see what I mean by 'no way back'.

In fact, in all ways this is a positive rather than a negative experience. I will feel good, feel healthy, look good, live longer and have more energy. And I won't have given anything up!

However, it wasn't all plain sailing. There were some shocks in store and that may also be the case for you. Be brave. There were quite a number of shocks for me when I filled in my food diary. Here are a few examples of what I used to eat. These were average days and at the time I did not think them excessive:

BREAKFAST:

Bowl of Chocolate Weetabix (150grams)	527 calories
Semi-skimmed Milk (170 ml)	123 calories
White Toast (4 pieces with Marmite)	417 calories
Butter (30 grams)	215 calories
Coffee with semi-skimmed milk (50ml)	25 calories
Croissant	272 calories
TOTAL	**1,579 calories**

SNACK:

Bag of Crisps	170 calories
Mars Bar	260 calories
TOTAL	**430 calories**

LUNCH:

Bacon and Sausage Sandwich	532 calories
Chips	640 calories
Galaxy Chocolate Bar	179 calories
Latte from Coffee Shop	250 calories
TOTAL	**1,601 calories**

AFTERNOON SNACK:

Starbucks Latte	250 calories
Krispy Kreme Donut:	220 calories
TOTAL	**470 calories**

DINNER:

2 cheese sandwiches	767 calories
Crisps	170 calories
Cake	150 calories
Nuts	177 calories
TOTAL	**1,264 calories**

SUPPER:

2 slices Marmite toast	332 calories
Coffee with semi-skimmed milk	25 calories
TOTAL	**357 calories**

Breakfast	1,579 calories
Snack	430 calories
Lunch	1,601 calories
Afternoon Snack	470 calories
Dinner	1,264 calories
Supper	357 calories
DAILY TOTAL	**5,701 calories**

I was utterly amazed. I knew that I was eating a little bit too much and probably not the right things, but how on earth was I eating not far off 6,000 calories a day when the only thing all the health books seemed to agree on was that I should eat 2,500?

For me, numbers always create understanding. Lord Kelvin once said ***"if you can't measure it in numbers, you don't truly understand it"***. Well, I now had the ugly truth in numbers and I was finally getting the picture. I was eating too much! Way too much! At last I was beginning to create a simple world where I understood my food and how it was affecting my weight. Before, I had not worried about the what, the how or even the type of food I was consuming, but finally the simplicity of the connection between calories and excess fat was beginning to dawn. It had taken a while but finally it was sinking in.

Before we move forward I hope you don't mind me giving you a quick summary of the important points we've covered and also some new insight into what to do to ensure success thus far.

1. Be clear on why you are going to get control of your weight. Health, kids, looks ...all of the above and more. The motivation really does not matter, so long as it's personal. Write it out and put it somewhere you can see it. Pin it on the door of the fridge, or next to your bed or anywhere that YOU see it often.
2. Calculate your true Body Mass Index (BMI). Just be honest and know what you need to lose to get down to a BMI of just below 25.00.
3. Give up giving up! Do not see this as a diet but as a change in your lifestyle. This is the NEW YOU not a temporary giving up of bad habits. Yours is now a positive world and anything with a negative feeling is hereafter forbidden.
4. Take control! Only you decide what goes in your mouth, not anyone else! If you eat it, it is your choice.
5. Get an App. like 'MyNetDiary'. It is available from iTunes or online for any PC including the one at your library and can be used free. Some versions are free

some are at a cost, but hunt around and find the best App. for you! If you can afford the paid version, I would recommend it, as the extra options are helpful but they are not essential. In the interest of fairness, I need to say right now "Other weight loss Applications and programmes are available".

6. Buy a set of scales to weigh food to the nearest gram. They are very affordable and utterly essential. If you think you can guess the weight, you are wrong! Scales don't have to be expensive so even if you're a bit strapped for cash, I promise in the nicest way; it will be the best £5 you EVER spend.

7. Spend one week recording everything you eat before you decide what to do going forward. Know the scale of the mountain you're about to climb.

8. If you cheat and do not write everything down, (what you eat, what you weigh and your measurements), you will fail to lose weight so this is really a waste of time. Please, please do not do it. I promise you it is better for you to know when you've had a bad day than kid yourself it really was not too bad.

9. If you've not got any pictures of yourself carrying all the excess flab you're intending to lose then get a few taken now, right at the beginning of the journey.

10. Remember that this is the last of the "tough love" advice you will need to give yourself. Every step forward from now on, knowing where you are and where you're headed is positive and will result in a lighter you.

I implore you - please do not skip these steps in understanding the scale of the issue. Nothing makes me more proud, now that I am stable with my weight, than to know I stared this problem in the eyes and beat it once and for all. Trust me you will feel exactly the same when you succeed.

Chapter Five
Help! I Need Somebody

More is less!
Losing weight alone is tough! Why? Because you will need to find all of the self-discipline on your own, with little or no encouragement. This was my observation on the first few days of the programme. I knew what I wanted and why I wanted it but I had not looked at any of the practical issues.

Lisa and I have two delightful children. One is a vegetarian, one is fussy. I was on a programme to lose weight and Lisa was a happy size 12 and not in need of losing anything, including her mind! All this added up to FOUR different meals for each meal time. I know this is a common issue for parents and we were no different but it did make life a bit tricky. Lisa decided to join me on our new programme. *This really made a difference and I believe that Lisa joining me on the journey was a key moment*.

Firstly it made the practicalities of making salads and healthier meals far easier as we were making them for two – at least now we were only providing THREE menu options per mealtime. Secondly, on the days I was feeling a little less enthusiastic, Lisa could help me through. However, what I also discovered was that, in addition to concentrating on my new life, I also gained huge positive energy by being able to support her. Somehow, by giving Lisa encouragement I seemed to absorb it into myself and it led me to this important conclusion....When trying to lose weight, *having a buddy with whom you can share the journey makes the whole thing many times easier.*

If you have a partner, try to get them engaged in the programme as possible. They may not need or want to lose weight but they can actively help you. If you do not have a partner who can support you, another alternative is to try to get a friend involved.

My own personal Facebook support team
I am truly blessed to have many friends. As a life time member of The Salvation Army I have pals all over the world. Canada, Australia and the USA are all represented and

I am privileged also to have friends in many parts of the UK and Europe. In addition, I have a great group of local buddies ranging from the parents of friends of the children and the school gate mums (I am in that group too) to some of my closest work colleagues. Facebook is a place where all of these different people in the different parts of my life see one single version of Jeremy. There have been times in my life when I would not have been too happy for all these groups to see the same story. Did I want "work" people seeing my trivial chat with my non-work friends? Social media raises many questions, this one among them. However, I have started to use my Facebook life to ensure that I am one single constant Jeremy, genuine and consistent. I don't try to be one person for one group of people and an entirely different Jeremy for another set of friends. It is a very peaceful place to be.

So my next thought was "how can I use this great support team to help me succeed?" I decided to put some status updates on my social media sites, mainly on Facebook, to my 400 or so friends. I wanted support, I needed support and I needed the positive energy that my friends would freely give me. It was part of the honesty we spoke about earlier. The more people knew about my intention to lose weight and keep it off, the more support I was likely to get.

Since the time I have started to post my weight status on Facebook, I have seen several others in that group now also start losing weight. A couple of my friends have even dared to do the same but in addition have publicly declared online their starting and target weights! I was not quite ready to do that!! But I was keen to put myself in a place where failure, if it happened, would be public. In a safe environment, namely with my friends, I wanted to ensure that I had the extra discipline of making a public statement and facing the consequences if I did not deliver. I still wanted to give myself the "positive handrails" and motivation of knowing that I did not want to fail in front of my friends and family. The two friends who put their numbers out in public are using exactly the same positive handrail.

Every time I lost 10lbs I was so excited to be able to update my status and to tell everyone I had dropped the weight and I received literally dozens of positive comments. "Well done, you look great" right through to "About time Fatty" from one buddy! In addition, I did not want to make it too easy for me to slip back up in weight. These announcements made it far harder to be tempted to go back. Losing weight was now a public activity and not a private battle.

Honesty with friends and family

At the same time as I mention positive engagement with friends and family, I need to share a slightly harder reality. Family were used to the old me. What follows is a perfect example of what I mean and I hope you can make the connection to relationships that you might have.

I am blessed with wonderful parents and they have been nothing but the best support in my life. Whenever I have been through tough times I KNEW I could rely on them without question. They love me deeply, this I know. It was that love which, for most of the last 15 years, led them to some very gently made comments:

"You need to look at your weight, my boy"

"How's your weight doing?"

"You're looking a little heavier, son".

I was always grateful that they cared, and enjoyed telling them "I have lost 2lbs" or some other comment that was a polite version of "I know I'm getting heavier and leave me alone". But their gentle persistence was appreciated. I am exactly the same in my gentle nagging, in love, of my children. It is what caring parents do.

However, at the same time over all those years, whenever I popped in to see my Mum and Dad, I was offered chocolate biscuits. Marks and Spencer's finest, large 'tea cakes' with a marshmallow inner and chocolate outer, or chocolate digestive biscuits. Divine! I soon realised that while I was making progress in my own home I needed those who were my friends and family to get onboard and not put temptation in my way. Soon I had a quick word with my parents and asked if they could help me by NOT offering these treats to me. After a few laughs, and a bit of teasing, the message was clearly delivered and received. We are a team, and while we have our different ways of getting to the best destination, we got there. I am sure that this conversation in a different house would look different, and I rejoice in the fact that different families have their own way of handling family business.

Just to be balanced, I needed help from my in-laws as well. They live in Guernsey in the Channel Islands, and island life is far more based around eating than most existences in the UK. My mother-in-law serves meals by putting the food on the table and you take what you want! It is a wonderful time for family. Meals are long and we talk, debate, laugh and argue while picking up the next cake. I find that type of grazing meal hard to handle. I love food and food loves me and when, in heated argument with my father-in-law, the next cake has been eaten yet I have not even noticed.

So, I spoke to my lovely in-laws to explain that from now on I will be taking a plate of food and then trying not to eat anything else but that which I planned to eat. I asked if we could have skimmed milk in the house for me. Guernsey full cream milk is a delight but these were calories I could ill afford. I eat lots of yogurt when on the island, and these are always in the fridge for me. I am sure you get the picture. I am trying to control this grazing aspect of my eating by making it as familiar as I can. I try to make sure that where possible I eat food that I know well and understand in calorific value. In many ways, I try to eat the same when in Guernsey as I do when at home.

It is working. Having recently returned from my last trip to Guernsey, I have come home 1lb lighter rather than the more normal outcome which is an increase of 4 to 5lbs! I will cover this ability to enjoy food even on special occasions in greater detail in the section on "birthdays and celebrations" and I do recommend you read that chapter if this has been an issue for you, as you may find a few tips that make holidays and occasions where you might have previously eaten excessively a far easier experience whilst still having fun.

Reaching your ideal weight is not a popularity contest
I have to be honest and say losing weight does not always make you popular with all of your friends. Through this experience I've found that for every one who is pleased for you, you will find another who at some level appears jealous and will start to make disparaging remarks.

The reality of today's world is that far too many people are overweight or obese. Deep down most of us know this fact, both on a personal and societal level, but we struggle to find the solution to our weight and the answer to the problem of how we will become healthier. When YOU start to succeed it will be only natural to have a few people feel slightly upset that it is not happening to them. I certainly would not worry about it but it is worth noting that the effect on some of your friends might be unexpected. Be warned.

So how to approach friends who also struggle with weight? I've been very open with them about my personal fears and weaknesses and that can help. In truth, I can't think of a way of being more open that writing this book. I have sensed that some of the "jealousy" has come from a fear that the next step when a friend has lost weight will be judgment for others who have NOT been able to get thinner. Nothing could be further from my personal feelings on this vital subject. I am now permanently there as a resource and encouragement for my friends if they want to talk, but now I am at my target weight I no longer post status updates on my personal Facebook page, I do not rub it in by constantly extolling the virtues of healthy living, I just live a wonderfully happy life with my friends and if they want me to help, they know where I am.

After a few tricky conversations around the time when I had dropped about 30lbs and was obviously thinner, I think I have repaired all my friendships back to their former glory. I've stopped worrying about comments like "You don't look well" or "'Have you been ill?" Instead of getting uptight I worked to restore the friendships which could have been seriously damaged by such remarks and made a deliberate check to ensure if I was at a good place with all my buddies. I did not ignore working at friendships but concentrated on building the relationships. I was getting huge support from my mates and I needed to give support to others who found my journey hard to watch.

On the subject of help, I found reading to be a wonderful assistance to me. Those people who know me well know that I had a good "grammar school" education, have been fairly successful at work, and yet I stand before you ashamed to admit that before I started my weight loss programme I knew so little about what made good healthy food choices.

Obtaining this information has changed my life for the better and it is a real disappointment to me that I was not aware of it earlier in my time on earth. I do not blame anyone but myself for this hole in my knowledge.

I have learned many things about many subjects over the years and simply chose not to find out about this critically important issue. My head has been full of all sorts of rubbish and although this information made me a deadly quiz competitor it didn't help when my ever expanding girth prohibited me from climbing trees with my family! I recommend that you learn about food groups.

Later I will include an "idiot's guide" to what I found useful but I thought it worthwhile mentioning it here, because we are in the section entitled "Help!"

Here are some questions for me and you related to help:

1. Who can I enlist to help me in this task?
2. What areas of my life will present situations where I am at risk of eating poorly?
3. What do I need to do to mitigate those risk areas?
4. Have I got a plan of action which will help me through the hard times? Write a short plan for each area and be intentional about how you can manage each specific issue. Keep it simple and do not include too many actions for any likely situation.

On this final question, I identified several areas and the few (3 or 4) things I was going to do to make life easier in tricky food environments. I have included a sample just so you can see one of my high level plans.

Family visits

1. Ask the family to be aware of my changed lifestyle and to help me by having available lower calorie food which I enjoy.
2. Make sure I let my family know what those foods might be, to make it easier for them when they shop.
3. Thank them before and after each visit for supporting me on this really important lifestyle change.
4. Ensure that I also eat some higher calorie food. A balanced healthy way of life includes treats and also proves to the family that I've not gone completely mad.

It worked perfectly!

Chapter Six
Operation Thinner

Well done for getting this far. By now you should have done a whole lot of thinking about why success is so important in your weight loss adventure. You should understand why you want to take control of your life and a little more about your relationship with food. You should hopefully have a clear image of what you will look like when you've lost the unwanted pounds, and what you want to feel like when you cross the finishing line!

Now it is time to live in your new world and start the journey. In this next chapter I am going to explain THREE vital aspects of your new world, nothing scary but really important. For this next stage you will need the following:

- A set of **DIGITAL bathroom scales** which operate to decimal places.
- A set of **DIGITAL kitchen scales** weighing to the nearest gram.
- **A MyNetDiary App. or similar App.** on your PC or Mobile device. Please see the link at the end of the book if you need to download this system.

I can already hear you saying "he hasn't mentioned new bathroom scales before!" You are correct but I now want to explain why I believe this was so important for me and helped me to succeed.

Measuring my behaviour not my weight
I had a nice set of old fashioned spring type scales that sort of pointed to a place on a circle when I stepped on them. In truth they were somewhat useless because if I didn't like what I saw when I looked down at the gauge I could move the arrow depending on how I leaned. If you have a set of these, you'll know what I'm talking about.

You see, the old me had a relationship with food which involved cheating. I knew I was cheating, I knew it was madness, but I would cheat nonetheless. I even used to try to weigh myself on carpet because the scales weighed me as a few pounds less than I registered when the scales were place on a tiled floor. For those of you who are smiling at this point, I know...it sounds ridiculous. We are all as bad as each other aren't we?

However, to master this weight loss palaver, I needed to KNOW what I weighed. A vague feeling of approximation is a poor substitute. This is a really important learning point. I had to stop cheating!

The golfer, who takes shots off her score at the end of the round, is not only cheating the people she is playing with but is also cheating herself. The fisherman who caught a whopper that slipped off the line before anyone else had a chance to see it or measure the record-breaking size is not only deluded and lying to others, but he is also cheating himself. The man who stole a Bass from a local pet shop and entered it into an angling competition was just cheating himself. The runners who tell people they completed a race faster than they really did, are not just lying but are also cheating themselves. There are many examples in life.

I needed to understand that when it came to food and weight loss I was not deceiving others by leaning on the scales to make them move, just myself. I had to learn to stop this. No diet will cure this issue. *A diet to which you do not adhere will not help you lose weight. Read that again please. A diet that you do not stick to will not help you lose weight because you are cheating!*

This is one of the many reasons why I believe, as do many others, that diets do not work, because they are so easily cheated on. This new programme and new way thinking was all about me understanding my weaknesses and taking actions to help me get stronger. It was about me changing my actions long term to get a different outcome. DIGITAL scales give you an exact number and there is no room for debate, and you will be tempted to debate unless you are superhuman, and I certainly am not! The digital scales should also give you a degree of accuracy, down to decimal places, and that's also important.

Why have scales that measure so accurately?
My bathroom scales are by Salter and cost me £15 and again for fear of plugging just one product I'll say it ....other makes are available. My scales show me my weight to an accuracy of 0.2lb. I can see the weight by pounds, or view it in stones/pounds or kilos and each to a great level of accuracy. A whole pound is a very large amount of weight to lose and during the programme we want to celebrate success. Trust me, losing even a little bit of weight is brilliant progress and you need to be able to see it on the scales and record it on your Application. If you think about it, you could have lost nearly half a pound in a week and if you've got scales which round up or down to the nearest pound, your success won't show up at all. I would have been sad if that

had happened because for me, every little loss was important. I wanted and I needed to see the scales showing me making progress. Small progress is still progress and if I was getting my eating and exercise behaviour under control, I had every right to be able to see it in the results. I recommend you take every opportunity to get all the positive messages that you possibly can. A set of digital scales is a brilliant way to spend £15 and will be well worth the money.

Why take the time to record everything?
As I have said before, this book is not about reinventing diets. There are hundreds of weight loss food programmes you can choose from and use their specific scientific information if that's what you wish to do. My heart is to set you up to succeed in whatever way you choose to take control of your size.

There is some basic information about food intake and weight loss which we all need to understand. Sorry to all you "old hands" at diets if this is all familiar territory for you but I know there will be some diet virgins reading this who may not be aware of the following. One of the most consistent pieces of information I saw when starting on my journey was that the average man needs approximately 2,500 calories a day and the average woman needs approximately 2,000. Now, I don't know about you but I am not average! And I really didn't understand what calorie intake was all about. Yet when I put my details into my chosen Application, I discovered a clear simple resource to help me figure it all out and to help me with my targets. MyNetDiary took my height and weight and activity level and gave me two important numbers. The first was the number of calories my body needed if I simply lay in bed all day and just breathed. These are the 'background calories' I need for my heart to pump, brain to tick and blood to be produced, all of the typical bodily functions. The second number was the amount of calories I would need to maintain my existing weight which at the time was, as I've explained, much greater than I wanted. The reason this information was so key to me was because I needed to understand a few important truths and to act accordingly. Having seen those numbers and recovered from the shock, I came up with 10 truths which I had to face up to and which motivated me.

TRUTH ONE – The more I eat the heavier I will be
This sounds so basic but for so many of us it is not in the front of our minds. For most of the population this is true, and it certainly included me. Unless I suddenly and hugely increased the amount of exercise I undertook, if I put more than 3,000 calories a day into my mouth, I would continue to gain weight. If I ate less I would get lighter.

We have all heard the stories of Olympic rowers eating 6,000 calories a day. Please ignore them all unless you are an Olympic rower. You have seen my open admission earlier and I was eating nearly 6,000 calories a day, so was it any wonder that I was getting heavier each and every year?

TRUTH TWO – Exercise is good for me
Exercise helps a great deal, but if you think you can still eat thousands of extra calories and lose it all in the gym, you had better be that Olympic rower! In my case, I soon worked out that unless I cut my food intake significantly I could run and row 10 hours a day and still be getting larger.

As time progressed and my fitness levels increased, I knew I could run for 30 minutes and burn up around 250 calories, so on days when I am going out to celebrate I use exercise as a super way of being able to have a dessert! However, I never allow myself to claim more than 500 calories of extra food because I don't want to have a life where, in order to indulge and eat what I want, I need to spend 13 hours of every day at the gym. I want nice food AND a life outside of the gym and apart from anything else, I need to go to work and spend time with my loved ones.

TRUTH THREE – You can start gradually
Chances are that when you start to read this book, you will be too heavy for your ideal weight. The good news is that when you calculate the number of calories to maintain your weight it will NOT be as low as 2,500 for men or 2,000 for women. This is because it's hard work being overweight and it takes constant feeding to stay at that overweight level. What it does mean for the overeater who is adding ounces every day, is that if you just started to eat the recommended number of calories, namely, 2,500, you would start to get thinner. In my case, I needed to eat nearly 3,000 calories simply to stay at my starting weight.

TRUTH FOUR – Losing a pound of fat is not luck, it is intentional
A pound of fat is lost when you manage to reduce your calorie intake by approximately 3,500 calories from the level needed to maintain your weight. Some say 3,600 but I use 3,500 to make the mathematics easier. In simple language, this meant that when I wanted to lose 1lb of fat per week and given the fact that I needed to eat 3,000 calories a day to maintain my weight, I worked out the simple sums and concluded that I had to do the following:

Given that 3,500 calories a week is equal to 500 a day (7 x 500 calories = 3,500 calories) if I cut my daily calorie intake to 2,500 (3,000 = the number needed to maintain my weight less 500, which is enough to lose one pound a week) I would get smaller! One pound at a time! Alternatively, I could choose to eat the proposed amount (3,000 calories) and daily exercise enough to burn up 500 calories. Whichever course I took I could achieve the same result. Miraculously that is exactly what happened!

So the great news is this. To lose weight I actually needed to reduce back to 2,500 and not 2,000 calories as I had expected. I was convinced that I would need to go under the normal 2,500 calorie daily intake for a man in order to lose weight. What a relief. It was BRILLIANT NEWS! *This is one of the simple pieces of logic I wish I had been taught at school!*

TRUTH FIVE – Have a target and don't go too fast

It is not a great idea to lose weight too quickly. This is a classic piece of advice to weight watchers and over the years I have found it to be very true. If you lose weight fast the chances of the flab reappearing are higher. However, I think I now know why this is the case. Diets – depriving you of food - do NOT exist in my world. It is now all about sustainable levels of eating. To lose lots of weight quickly, you need to virtually starve and as soon as you return to any sense of normal you will start to increase your food intake and as a result you will increase your weight. This added to the body's natural metabolism becoming far less effective when you starve yourself, means you may be in trouble if you lose weight too fast. Please try to be patient. Small is good in this game. I lost at approximately 2lbs a week for the whole programme and I do not think you should consider going faster without significant medical reason or advice. When you read chapter 7 please take this advice seriously. If you do try to lose weight faster, please make sure you are in regular contact with your Doctor or GP.

I know you will be eager to get going and start dropping pounds immediately but I would suggest you plan your loss to be a little slower than you actually desire. You will feel a great deal more satisfied being ahead of a plan at 1lb per week than you will if you find yourself behind by 2lbs a week. Remember, positive inputs at all times!

TRUTH SIX – In time you will eat less than you do now

The lighter you get, the fewer the number of calories you will require, so will you need to go back to the weight loss plan from time to time as you lose the pounds. Sorry about this, but it is true. In my new weight, I now need 2,500 calories per day to maintain my lower weight, and not the 3,000 that I required when I was so much heavier. My body does not have to work as hard just to live and breathe. It does not have to fight to keep my heart beating and ensure all my vital organs are working, so it needs less basic energy. The same will be true for you just as it has been for both Lisa and me. However, on a positive note I am so motivated to stay the same (smaller) size and I have learned what foods help me stay fuller for longer, I now really don't feel tempted to eat more very often.

TRUTH SEVEN – I will not put on weight if I have a bad day
I am now very focused on my weekly calorie intake. If I have a bad day and eat lots, it is normal and not the end of the world. In fact, on my last trip to Guernsey I went out with Lisa for a huge meal at a lovely hotel and still came home at the end of that holiday with my mother-in-law, including a number of birthday celebrations, lighter than when I got on the plane. In fact, I'd go so far as to recommend that you need "Bad Days" once in a while, just not every day!

TRUTH EIGHT – Calorie counting is easy these days and it works
Counting calories has undoubtedly worked for me as a long term way of losing weight. It is most certainly not the only way of losing weight but it has worked in my case. I have struggled with other systems, but not because they do not help me lose weight, in fact several I have encountered worked really well. *My problem has always been how to transition from the 'diet phase' back to the 'normal life' phase.* I have found it impossible to go out for work meals and try to use 'points' or 'syns' or one of the many other variants. I know people who have cracked that but as I said earlier, this calorie system worked really well for me. I can keep a good mental note of what I can eat and manage to remain stable. You see, I want a life including ALL foods, not just some. I want a normal life where I have a positive relationship with ALL the foods I eat. I want a way to compare which foods are good for me and which less good, so that I can chose what I do eat and what I don't eat. Calorific information has given me this flexibility. I found it easy and with practice, I believe you could also find it simple.

TRUTH NINE- Only eat food you LOVE
I now have a policy of only eating food I really enjoy. If I take a bite and don't like something, I leave it. If I love it, I eat it. Why would I choose to waste precious calories on foods I do not like? I even apply this to brands of food that I know I like. As an example, I eat lots of Mullerlight Yoghurts. I love them. I do not say they are the best but they are my yoghurt of choice. If they are available I eat them, if not I do try other yoghurts. However, if I find them simply not as nice, rather than

eat something I don't like, I will stop and wait till I can have something that I enjoy. Follow your instincts.

TRUTH TEN – The Spice Girls are the answer
Some friends have accused me of being far more disciplined than they could ever be. This is nonsense. I've just learned to focus. At work, I often tell people the secret to projects is answering "The Spice Girls Question". The song "Wannabe" has brilliant words. "So tell me what you want, what you really, really want". My view is simple. In this game, there are lots of "Wannabes". The reason the visualisation is so important is that you need to know not just what you want ("I want to be thin"), but what you "really, really want." The more detail you have on the lower levels of what you want, the easier it is to focus on what you "really, really, want."

I guess my experience shows me that the gap I originally had in my head and in my subconscious was an understanding of what it was I REALLY wanted. Well, I now tell you this - I want a long healthy, fit, fun life a heck of a lot more than I want a Full English Breakfast every day. I want my new clothes to fit tomorrow a lot more than the bag of crisps I fancy today. It just comes down to motivation and choices about what I want in my life.

Digital kitchen scales
At the start of this chapter when I listed the three vital aspects of your new weight loss world, the second required item was my Digital Kitchen Scales. When I began the programme I tried a great game and I recommend it to anyone. It is easy, so get a bowl and try to measure out the recommended portion of All Bran Cereal, or any other Cereal for that matter, into that bowl. The first time I tried my portion was over 100grams, which is a shame as the recommended amount per portion of the Cereal I used is 50grams! If I used just my "expert eye" to measure my food portion I would have under reported my calories by a factor of 50%. What's the likelihood that I would then have complained that the calorie counting was not working and diets are rubbish. In fact, I would have gone into my usual "why bother?" cycle, convincing myself, yet again that "I can't lose weight, dieting is for others but not me!", "I am a victim blah, blah, blah".

The cost of avoiding this fundamental problem is around £3.99 for a set of kitchen scales that measure to the nearest gram. When I was starting to lose weight I would have to say this was one of the best investments I made. To this day, Lisa and I weigh everything we can. I now laugh when I think back to my previous arrogance at thinking that I could, naturally and without any help or particular knowledge, know exactly what 50grams of this or 100grams of that looked like, and what the calorie content would be. Every cook book recommends the amount of each type of ingredient for a successful meal, yet we do not carry on the same behaviour when it comes to writing down calories by weight. Strange really, but this is another behaviour I have learned to change.

Before I end this section, I do want to confess that I still do eat some really bad stuff. Sometimes I am amazed I lost weight, at all. But I eat "bad stuff" by choice. I plan the whole day's or whole meal's food in advance and if I want a 'naughty' dessert, then I eat a lighter main course, or a smaller lunch that day. I think more consciously about it. I make informed, balanced decisions about what I consume. So when I eat "bad stuff", I eat it in a good way! I am intentionally in control, and I am still at the weight I desire. In view of the ten truths listed here, there's no list of questions this time round, but I would recommend you take a few minutes to check the truths again and see how they feel to you. How can you apply them to your experience?

Chapter Seven
Eating Less for Beginners

Having had such a pleasant surprise when I discovered how many calories I could eat for my new eating plan, I still needed to start reducing the amount I actually consumed. I want to be totally open with you about what I did and also what I would do if I were starting again, which I will not because I will never be my old weight again!

Around the time I was looking to finally take control of my weight I came across a website from a company called Evolution Slimming. They had a product called Liquid Diet Drops. I took these drops for the first FOUR weeks of my new regime. These drops involved a taking a small amount of the special liquid at the beginning of the day and 12 hours later. They had the effect of significantly reducing my hunger craving in those first few weeks. In addition to taking the drops, the scheme insists you go onto a very low calorie count (VLCC), which is effectively a very low carbohydrate eating programme. To put it into some context, a normal mid-range healthy food programme would include around 275 grams of carbohydrate but at this time I was down to less than 50 grams. To achieve this level I had to give up cereal, bread, pasta, sugar, rice and potato, in fact just about everything I enjoyed. While I don't recommend any scheme or protocol that focuses on one food group for any length of time, this diet claimed a few things:

- VLCC (500 calories a day) would help reset your metabolism.
- The drops would ensure you did not feel hungry.
- The drops would help you lose up to 1lb a day.

I was deeply cynical. Yet I did discover the following:

My fears that I could not reduce my food intake to that low level proved to be unfounded. Indeed, my metabolism did indeed reset as I have seen by the later results I have enjoyed. Amazingly, the drops did take away most of my hunger pangs. I cannot explain why, nor will I try to but even though I had to give up carbohydrates and focus more on proteins I managed to get through the day comfortably. It was during this time I learned to enjoy salads. These great foods are your friends for life and I will cover this more in Chapter 10 as well as in Appendix 1, where you can see some of my personal sample menus. Needless to say salads are bulky, do not take many calories, and are not properly carbohydrates as in they only have traces of carbohydrate in them, so in the context of this VLCC they are perfect.

As I have already mentioned, I only took the drops for four weeks. In that time I did not lose as much as a pound a day. However, I did lose 15lbs in those four weeks, so I achieved 0.5lb a day. Far more importantly, most days when I weighed myself I was lighter. This was a great motivator and I would say was actually the best thing about the LDD Protocol. I have never felt that success breeds success as deeply as I do now. My new lifestyle owes a lot to actually seeing I was making progress every single week. The fact that my first stone was gone was a great comfort but this LDD protocol was certainly not a sustainable way to live. However, if you are morbidly obese it still does not look a bad option.

The next challenge was how to stop taking the drops. I think in all of us there is a little rebel and we show it in many different ways as for me, I am not good at doing exactly what I am told. As a child I used to walk on the cracks in the pavement just because I could. I am sure we all do things throughout our life in a slightly individual way that might even be described as "quirky". At this point of the journey I took myself aside and gave myself a really strong talking to. It went something like this:

- For once in your life you are not going to ask why.
- You will follow the instructions, without question.
- Do not think you know best, you do not.
- You have done brilliantly well in getting so far, do not put all the weight back on again.

So I followed the LDD instructions to the letter. The first week after the drops, I increased my food intake to 1,200 calories. For that whole week I felt full and satisfied because I was in food heaven, having near trebled my food intake, and the drops were still in my system, suppressing my hunger. For the second week, I added one portion of carbohydrate a day. The first day was cereal. Oh how I had missed it, but I was strong and stuck to the instruction of only one portion.

It was during this time I started to feel the start of what I can safely call "hunger", and I certainly needed to be strong willed for a few days. However, my system was getting used to my new way of eating. On the third week, I started to add two portions of carbohydrate. The LDD scheme was very firm that if you just went back to full levels of carbohydrates you risked regaining all your lost weight. ***Now I learned a new discipline called compliance!***

After one final week of three portions I was able to go back to a full range of carbohydrates and to this day nothing is off the menu! I do keep an eye on my carbohydrate intake because nearly always if I put a pound back on it is because I have started to go back to my old ways of eating too many carbohydrates but again this is covered more fully in Chapter 10.

After 9 weeks I was free of LDD. As you see, it worked for me in those first few weeks but I admit I could not have coped with it for another single day. Many people go back for a second time but I have to say I could not do it again. Yet I will always be grateful for the experience and I want to explain in detail why I feel this way.

Compliance can be good for you

I have always been an individual and some may even say a maverick. As previously mentioned, just before I started with LDD I told myself that this was a new task and I really did not want to fail. I wanted to be certain that I had tried my very best.

At work I have been involved in many new training programmes on health and safety as well as financial matters. The world of money laundering and competition law is now one which I have to take very seriously indeed. Compliance at work is NOT optional. Yet in other places I have never truly felt comfortable doing as I was told. Something deep inside me told me I have a slightly better way to do things. However, as well as learning to comply with the LDD scheme I actually have learned a whole new series of skills around compliance and following processes that, surprisingly, haven't just helped in my weight loss but have also transferred to my career.

Why did I always feel the need to question nearly everything? Compliance, I now realise, is not a weakness but a huge strength. To all those I have ever questioned with an "I know better" mentality behind my question, I publicly apologise. Liquid Diet Drops was a good weight loss tool for me. Judge it by the numbers. I lost 15lbs in 4 weeks. However, I can't begin to quantify the wider benefits and skills that it taught me and these skills were to be VERY important later on in my weight loss journey.

The behaviours I learned

1.   **Know what I eat.** I had never really thought about an App. to help me before. I certainly never thought about the different brands of food having very different calorific values. Cheddar Cheese is Cheddar Cheese isn't it? Well, I learned that if you buy it right you can save 50%of the calories! By having to input the foods

into my App. I learned what to eat and now that I am far more informed, I am not the same person.

2. **Make choices.** I now choose what I eat. No one does that for me. This is now true in every area of my life. I choose if I exercise, I choose if I put my clothes away, I choose if I take care in my appearance. I choose if I put others before me. Life is about choices, but it was only when I tackled my weight and I had proof that in the past I did not make very good choices when it came to food, that my mind opened up this thinking in other areas of my life.

3. **Discipline.** I needed discipline not to cheat. I needed discipline to be honest. I needed discipline to plan the right foods. So many areas of my life now experienced a more disciplined Jeremy. I did not have discipline and then lost weight. I found discipline through commitment to losing weight.

4. **Exercise makes me less stressed.** When I am having a tough time at work, I should be able to take time to relax and stay fit. I cope with stress better now I am thinner.

5. **I am less driven to win arguments.** I have developed a far greater quietness and calmness. I am more able to win the war than fight the battle. No longer do I have to question everything and I am far more content.

6. **No objective is out of reach.** In every aspect of my life I look for challenges. I always wanted to write a book, and wondered what I could write about. I know the best place to start is with the things you know something about. What did I know about which was any use at all to the wider world? Well, I now know about losing weight! You are reading the proof that I have attained a key objective in life, with some help from a few brilliant friends. I now have new focus on achieving things, and a quiet inner belief I CAN deliver on every one of them.

All in all, not bad for a few drops I would say!

The anti-LDD lobby will tell you that you will lose the same amount of weight by cutting to 500 calories and you do not need to spend money on the drops. They may be right, I really do not know because I took the drops. Maybe the placebo effect was at play and I was not hungry as my head thought it was taking anti-hunger drops? Who knows? Lisa, my wife, lost about the same amount also by taking the LDD drops, and we have had several friends decide to try the same route and it has worked for all of them. So it appears something is working, somewhere, somehow.

You will recall that I mentioned at the beginning of this chapter that I might have done it differently if I did it again.

So now I admit that, given my time over, I may well have grasped the nettle at the very beginning and NOT used hunger suppressants. It is a bit like a mother who opts for an epidural during childbirth. The help was there and I took it, but now I wonder what it would have been like if I had not used it. I guess I am a "take the help that is there" kind of a guy!

But as you know, I lost 15lbs with drops and 55lbs using my new behaviours without them. Even though I took the drops, I learned new skills through that period which have lasted long beyond that initial month.

Watching what I eat and how much I exercise is the absolute key. I had approximately 70lbs to lose and was pretty scared it was an impossible task. I thought about how I could make it easier. LDD definitely worked and I am pleased it worked, but with what I know now, I am not certain they were necessary. I am a passionate advocate of not focusing on individual food groups and I do admit that LDD does appear to be against that base principle. I now know I could have made it without the drops and I know you can make it without them too. So to summarise, if you decide to try LDD as a protocol, know if you follow the plan it will work. However, if you can stick to the content included in the following chapters on how I lost the other 55lbs, you will equally succeed.

I have two additional things I need to say before finishing this section. Do not, under any circumstances start to exercise when still on a VLCC protocol. You simply do not have enough energy or calorific intake to handle it. I tried, and can confirm it is a bad idea! Just for the record, I tried not knowing it was a bad idea and it was only when I looked it up on the internet that I realized my mistake! Secondly, it is worth noting that Lisa and I are not aligned on LDD and my personal conclusions. She is far more on the side that LDD made the biggest difference in resetting her metabolism. She took the drops for only three weeks not four and since she came off them and followed the same method as I described of a gradual build up in her carbohydrate intake, has managed to stay firmly fixed at her new weight and size with seemingly little difficulty but a significantly different way of life.

Chapter Eight

Fit

One of the downsides of being too large had to be that I never really felt that comfortable in a gym. One of the few things I have tried as many times as dieting has been joining a gym and it has been a cycle of disasters. I would pay a joining fee, then go twice and get discouraged and finally not visit the place again. I was far too busy, or so I would tell myself. How many others can tell variants of the same story? Far too many, I fear.

The big chap in the gym
Let's take a step back into the recent past. I am a pleasant 6ft- tall man who sadly weighs nearly 18 stone and sports a 42 inch waistline. Most men with a 42 inch waist will remember how upsetting it was when a 38 inch trouser size turned into a 40 inch. I am sure that most women have exactly the same feeling when size 18 clicks into size 20. I held firm for a few years before I gave in to 42 inch and I was worried it would never stop. Size made me self-conscious and going to the gym was a potential nightmare. I imagined everybody (not some people but everybody) would watch and stare at the large chap who got tired and sweaty and generally made themselves look like a fool.

I mentioned earlier about the power of negativity in the whole process of weight loss and this is another great example of that. In reality, not a single person stared. Most people were too busy working on their own bodies to worry about mine! Perception and reality were very far apart. I want to use my next "Thank You" to the Village Hotel, in Maidstone, Kent. Lisa and I joined up on one of their special offers.

We decided that we needed the discipline of each spending a sum of money, which would be wasted if we did not attend and use the facilities.

There is a great story of a famous classical composer who always stayed in bed too long. However, his wife needed to change the sheets and he simply would not get up. In desperation she went to his piano and played an incomplete cadence (the last few notes of a piece). It grated on the musician so much that he simply had to get up and play the last chord. I know exactly how he felt. Spending £78 a month and not going to the gym would have grated badly. We were going and that was that! However, the folk at the gym at the Village made exercise seem like it was something normal, rather than something super people with no flab did to annoy us larger folks.

What makes a good gym?
At the hotel where we have our gym, we also have a pool, a dance studio, a spinning studio and lots of friendly people. We also have a Starbucks, a restaurant and a pub type bar, to tempt us as soon as we walk out! However, the most important aspect of the place is the staff and in addition to good staff you also need nice customers. I have been to several gyms where everyone is already fit, inhabiting a fit and thin world all their own where no one else matters. I hate that world, and still do even today.   A brilliant gym has customers of all ages. It also has customers of all sizes as well as both genders.

If you go to a gym and you cannot find anybody over 30 years of age or anyone trying to get fit and not there yet, the environment will be very competitive. My gym is simply brilliant. We all talk to each other. We all help each other. I have asked people in all parts of the establishment how they have got so fit and every time I received a positive response.   It is like a big family. We have the younger ones trying to get bigger muscles or fitter. We have the parents trying to lose weight, get fit, and relax. There are the grandparents staying healthy and dropping pounds. Our gym includes people of every shape and size. There are people who have been members of the club for years and people who have just joined. When you're looking for a good gym, I advise you to shop around and find one like ours and you will not go far wrong!

So, as I've said, I did not like gyms and I did not need many excuses to have a hissy fit and stop attending. The staff at my gym introduced themselves to me by actually explaining the way the place worked. They also explained all the strange machines, and what they did. The staff also took the time to help me understand the benefit to my overall health that each exercise group would bring.

I started with the rowing machines. I think the sitting down part appealed to me, but I found I could do rowing and not feel like I was going to die. I was also aware in the early days that there was a large mirror the whole length of the gymnasium. It was bad enough I felt large but did I really have to see myself sweat? Well, over time I grew to love those mirrors. I doubt I would have looked in a mirror much at home but over the weeks I started to see a real difference in what I saw, and I liked it. I had confronted my fear of seeing myself and now it was a real positive in my motivation. My confidence was growing and I even started to think I might wear a T-shirt that would actually show my shape!

I also remember starting to look forward to seeing if I could beat my best times. What was it with me and numbers? Do you remember I mentioned Lord Kelvin earlier and his quote on needing numbers to understand things? Well he was so right. I had got numbers into my life in a big way.

- What was my weight? A fact based number.
- What was my target weight? Another fact based number.
- How many calories was I eating each day? I went to my App. and got another number.
- How fast could I row 2,000 metres on the rowing machine? Yes! A Personal Best time!

I had managed to stop looking for excuses and found safety in facts and numbers. In fact, I was surrounding myself in numbers as I saw the new me evolving. Before the start of the programme, I hated the numbers I saw before me, because I did not like the honesty they brought into my life. Now, I was beginning to take control. I felt like Admiral James T. Kirk on the USS Enterprise. I was boldly going to new places. Although it wasn't the Starship Enterprise and I wasn't a member of the Star Trek crew I was in control of my ship and I was on the bridge with masses of instruments telling me everything I needed to know!

After a few weeks of visiting the gym, I needed some variety in my exercising, to add to my rowing. So I tried riding the exercise bike. I know what you're thinking - another sitting down machine but I was not ready to exercise standing up just yet! I found the static cycle really hard work. I had never owned a bike, even when I was a child, and as such I did not have the thousands of miles children build up in their little legs whilst permanently riding up and down the street or to school. After sticking at it for a few weeks I slowly got the hang of it. I even moved onto riding the posh bikes with screens up front, so I could ride through the French countryside. I started to watch the Jeremy Kyle show on the screens. I discovered sides to life that I never knew existed. The mind boggles!

Time to take a dip and get wet
I felt that I needed to add swimming to my list of movement. I have a shocking

swimming technique but something interesting happened when I moved to the pool.

Over many years I had taken the children to public swimming pools and as I was naturally short sighted I always had to wear glasses, at least until about 4 years ago. As I was larger than the average swimmer and my eyes were so bad that I had to wear my glasses in the pool I was very self-aware and felt I stood out from the crowd. But I feared I might fish the wrong kids out of the pool if I chose to leave them in the locker. That's leave the glasses in the locker room, not the children! For some reason, as yet unexplained to myself, a few years back I had laser eye surgery and had them fixed. This was most unlike me, as I am normally risk averse but it worked a treat and I could finally leave my glasses in the locker and the children of Maidstone could swim safely without risk of a semi-blind guy insisting it was time to go home. In my routine, I started to swim lengths of the pool. I needed to work out a time when I could go and use the lanes. I needed to plan and not just let it occur. I found a really good time to swim and made it happen. Gradually I was able to go from swimming one length to swimming two without stopping. Then I progressed to four lengths and more, and slowly I improved!

I found swimming very good for me both physically and mentally. The exercise benefits of swimming are well known but feeling that I was in a pool and happy to be in just my shorts was progress for me. I could feel it, and I was thrilled that all the life style changes were beginning to make sense. What had started as a vision of what I wanted for myself and my life was actually beginning to be delivered. I really felt good about myself. I nearly had to tell myself off for getting too complacent, but in fact I used it as a way to drive deeper into my new life.

After a while I found I had lost nearly two stones (28lbs) in weight, and I needed to buy a smaller set of swimming trunks. Another positive milestone! In most areas of life you can still wear clothes that are slightly too big, but please do not try that with swimming costumes! With the smaller trunks, the smaller belly and the ability to see, I found myself feeling far happier in this environment. I started to think "I can do this". What was so exciting was the "this" was applying to all sorts of new things. Swimming was now definitely fun! I will cover the whole aspect of shopping in Chapter 14 as I have masses of experiences to share in that space. So, just to keep some sense of order to this journey I will now stick to exercise-related feelings.

I had a few exercises I could do with some degree of competence, and I was feeling more energetic, the lighter I became, the thinner I got and I made a huge discovery.

I was no longer that worried about my weight, but was interested in my trouser size.

As I mentioned earlier, I was a 42 inch waist trouser when I set out on this journey and I knew people saw every single one of those 42 inches. I wanted to be a 32 inch waist but was that even remotely possible? I then remembered - I was in control of my life! So I made a note that while I would stick to my health related target of a BMI of under 25, I would not stop until I was a 32 inch waist. Lisa started at a UK dress size 12/14 and was now a regular size 10 all over. I was so proud of her as she had always wanted to be a size 10. Why is it women do this so well? She had shown me that even people who do not really need to lose that much weight can take control and achieve their long held size goals. In fact by the time we had finished Lisa had become a size 8 and was happier with her looks than she had ever been.

Later I will add my more advanced tips on exercise in a second 'getting fitter' chapter. This section is merely a focus on how I started on the road to enjoying exercise, and the environment I needed to make it successful.

As a final note I want to stress the subject of movement. In my experience, one of the keys to weight loss is just to keep moving. Walk! Walk as much as you can. I started to use a pedometer to count my steps. These little gadgets are cheap and easy to use but I was amazed at what I discovered. I commute into London and on those days I hit my daily target of 10,000 steps with ease. Somehow, moving around the office just adds up. However, on the days I work at home I was completing as little as 3,000 steps. The recommended number of steps for a given day is 10,000 and so at home I was only moving 30% of the amount I should.

So what might be the solution? When working at home, I go for a run at lunch, or go to the gym, or walk to the shop. I find a way to move. The company I work for is an active member of the Global Corporate Challenge, where we enter teams of 7 people into a league walking 10,000 steps daily for a period of 112 consecutive days. I joined a team and it really helped me with the self-discipline I required. Being part of a team meant I did not want to fail or let down my fellow team members. I took my pedometer on holiday and work trips and all-in-all I commend the discipline of movement to you with all of the passion I can muster.

I assure you that whilst I will not wear a pedometer every day of my life, I will make sure I have one around and take to measuring my steps every so often just to ensure I do not drop back into bad sloth-like immobile habits!

So it is time for the summary questions:

1. Where can I exercise?
2. Is there a good family gym which I can join nearby?
3. What exercise do I enjoy or who can I ask to help me with setting up a routine?
4. Do I have a pedometer? If not, I need one.
5. How many steps do I currently walk each day?
6. What can I do to increase the amount of walking I currently take? Can I park further from work or from the station or change my routine to build in more steps?
7. How would I feel seeing myself get slimmer?
8. When can I start?

Chapter Nine
Rewards

One step at a time

I do so vividly remember when I started out on this road that the overwhelming feeling that "70lbs is a large amount of weight to lose" was never too far from my mind. As a Project Manager, and I am used to undertaking large tasks that cannot be handled in one simple dash, so in every job I undertake at work, I break it up in to small bite-sized chunks. Years ago I was told you can't eat the elephant in one mouthful, and I now know it is true in every aspect of life. Big tasks need plans and they need milestones to head towards and to drive behaviour. Putting it simply, losing all my weight was going to be a long road and I needed to create a world of single steps and not worry about the length of the road. Every significant achievement in the history of the world has started with a single step. This book is my way of sharing with you some of the steps I took to help me on the long journey and I hope by now you are beginning to see that *the method of dieting is really not that important, it is the planning that makes it all come together.*

Milestones

When I am running one of my projects at work I will make sure I have special milestone meetings where we aim to have made a certain amount of progress by a certain time. These invariably have Senior Managers in the room and this is a great way of focusing the mind. So I needed to create the same sense of focus on my weight loss programme. Lisa was brilliant at buying into the concept of rewards. I wanted to have something to help me keep focused during the dark days and small rewards seemed like a good plan. Although she had far less weight to lose, Lisa was on the same journey as me and we were both able to come up with fun, and not always too expensive, ways of rewarding each other for continuing to lose weight.

Tough projects are rarely about building things. While things usually need to be built, the overriding challenge is to get the people involved and committed to the right behaviours. At work, encouraging people to hit deadlines, or attend meetings on time, or build and share a common vision of success is far harder than designing a new process. If nothing else, when you design a new process, it will not argue with you! The rewards part of our journey was not so much about the actual amount of weight lost but on rewarding the right behaviours that will keep Lisa and me healthy for the rest our lives.

The rewards explained

When I lost my first stone (14lbs) I was so thrilled when Lisa came home with a lovely new shirt for me. She had decided that my clothes were looking a little too big and wanted me to have something to fit the new me! It was a simple gesture, but one that helped me on two levels. First, on a practical level, I had a new shirt that fitted. However, on another level it also helped me to notice that even although I had lost only 20 per cent of my target, Lisa could already see a difference. If Lisa could see a difference, then others could also see a difference and the spring in my step was just a little bit more pronounced.

By the time I had lost another stone, I got a new jumper. It was winter and my size difference was beginning to become very pronounced. Oh how I loved the feeling that I was no longer in need of "Extra Large" Clothes. I had moved to a world where I was now into "Large" size in certain brands. This movement to a world that did not involve the word "Extra" was wonderful. I promised myself I would never again, from that date, buy an XL item of clothing from the high street shops, and I haven't.

Three stone gone was a bit of a fantasy feeling for me. I had never lost more than 20lbs in my life and so moving to a world where I had lost over 40lbs was very special. I was so looking forward to my reward. In the past, to mark something momentous, Lisa and I would have gone out to have a celebration meal but this time I was not expecting to do that.   However, I was wrong, totally wrong. We went out and ate. How great is that? I love the unexpected and this fell into that category. We had to be able to celebrate and eating out was going to be on our list of things to do for life. All it meant was we had a chance to practice our new behaviours in selecting better, more healthy options. I will discuss eating out and travel more thoroughly later in the book, but this first time was wonderful. Lisa looked amazing and I felt great. We were in a wonderful restaurant eating to celebrate being so much thinner and it felt suitably crazy!

Stone number four was time for a new jacket or coat. I went out into Maidstone and bought a new Hugo Boss coat. I love that coat! I also loved haggling over the price in the shop with the owner and needless to say the 60% discount helped me decide on this particular reward. I had never, ever bought designer clothes. Truth be told, they never made them in my size! Another new world was beginning to open up. It was not that designer clothes were an aspiration for me, but they represented a world from which I had previously been excluded.

Unexpected finish to my plan
For a hobby, I love playing the trumpet and I had always promised myself when I lost the final part of the 70lbs that I would buy a new trumpet. I never did, and I don't think I ever will. I am just so thankful for all the support, love and encouragement I've received, I don't need to be rewarded anymore. Just a quiet, humble prayer of rejoicing was all I needed. When I was listing some of the changes that had occurred in my life as a result of the programme, I was beginning to feel that losing the weight was just a side benefit and I had actually started to find the true me. I had always laughed that "inside me was a thin man, maybe two". Well, one of those two seemed to have disappeared and I had found the inner me that did not need a pat on the back!

I can't help but wonder what you would enjoy as a treat or reward on the journey? However, far more important to me is how you will feel the day you hit your target weight. For those of us who have spent a lifetime being overweight, I know that it is just such an amazing sensation that I am sure it will be all the reward we need. I bet at this exact moment you are thinking that it can't be you, that only other people have the self-control or discipline. This whole book is to say I understand that feeling. I walked that road and yet, amazingly, I took control and lost the lot, and so can YOU! YES, YOU CAN!

I am now in the privileged position of having had hundreds of people come up to me and ask how on earth I have lost so much weight. Helping others achieve the same or better has been without a doubt the best reward of the entire experience. When you succeed, you will affect so many others - your friends, your family, your work colleagues and even people you do not know that well, like customers or parents at the school gate. So, I will end this section by asking you only three questions:

1. How will it feel to think about so many others looking at YOU and being amazed at what YOU have achieved?
2. What rewards would you give yourself for each 10lbs you lose?
3. How will you feel knowing you helped others to lose weight by inspiring them with what you have achieved?

Chapter Ten
The Power of Salad

As I have said many times before in this book, I never wanted to go on a traditional diet. My fear had always been that if I did not change my eating habits, whatever weight I had lost would simply return. It was not a fear without experience. This issue had hit me every time I lost weight and I was determined that it would not catch me again. After lots of thinking I could only see one option. I had to rewire my thinking and so that is exactly what I did.

We've already seen that the widely accepted consumption of calories for your "average" man is 2,500 per day. The "average" woman comes in at 2,000. Now, 2,500 calories can be seen in two basic ways. Either it is a lot or it is not a lot. Perspective is a wonderful thing. That 2,500 when starting from 5,000, is a small number. However, that same 2,500, when seen against the 500 calories I was eating on the VLCC protocol, is sheer heaven! So you have a personal choice to make. I think I have mentioned several times that this is all about positive thinking as well losing weight. Therefore, you will not be surprised I chose to process my new calorific regime as "plentiful". I simply needed to look for a place where I could use my calories in such a way that I felt full and happy with what I was eating. My only question was - did such a place exist?

Salads have never really been a key part of my eating experience. I guess I simply could not get excited about lettuce. I know now that this was a big mistake and in truth I am upset I have wasted so many years without this wonderful natural food in my day-to-day diet. It was most certainly my loss! There are so many ways of making a salad and they have helped me revolutionise my culinary tastes.

As I got further into my new world I became aware from my iPad App. that the days I seemed not to lose any weight, or even slightly increase, were tied directly into the days I ate the most carbohydrates. *Being focused on numbers helped me see the trend* and so I started to work out ways of reducing my over dependence towards this food group. I also noted that when I was tired or stressed my first basic instinct was to reach for carbs. Crisps, pizza, and chips were always at the front of my mind - all heavy carbohydrate sources and all of them giving me a short term relief from my lack of energy or stress but also high in calories and low in nutritional value.

When I gave into this base behaviour I always struggled to eat within my calorie count. If you consider that most normal pizzas alone will contain well over one thousand calories, it is really not that surprising. When I had been on the VLCC of only 500 calories a day I had eaten lots of salads and they were a good way of eating low calories for a meal yet feeling full for a long time. I was wondering why I had stopped eating the green stuff when I had come through that regime? In truth, salads were easier when I was forbidden carbohydrates, but I was seeing that when I had a choice I wanted all the bad stuff! After some soul searching I started to use my salads as a way of having one meal a day that took up very few calories. This gave me the flexibility to eat nearly whatever I wanted in the other two meals, as long as I had sensible portion sizes. I will openly confess to you that I have to remind myself of this even now. These pesky carbohydrates will keep popping back into my normal long term diet and I will always have to keep them under control.

From a personal perspective, and without any medical training, I do not feel comfortable with any medium or long term focus on one particular food group. I have many friends who focus on eating nearly all their calories from protein and I feel as uncomfortable with the long term effects of that as I would do in banning the carbohydrates which we need for many different bodily functions. It is all about balance. *My issue is a personal temptation to over balance toward carbohydrates, and I have to be very intentional in making sure I fight what for me is now destructive behaviour.*

I now eat so many types of salad both at home and in restaurants. I want to give you an idea of the scope I currently eat just to demonstrate that it is far from boring as a long term way of eating.

My basic salad will **ALWAYS** contain:
Lettuce, tomato, cucumber

It will **OFTEN** contain combinations of:
carrot, egg, bacon, cress, grapes, strawberry, apple, mango, orange, parmesan cheese, cottage cheese, feta cheese, gouda cheese, small bacon bits, chicken, turkey, tuna, ham, fish fingers, walnuts, almonds, sweetcorn, peas, plain pitta chips.
Dressings now include balsamic vinegar, low fat caesar, low calorie mango, lower fat mayonnaise.

It will **RARELY** contain:
Cheddar cheese, blue cheese, full fat mayonnaise.

There are so many options available. I love to add fruit to my salad with a good protein source like chicken. Lisa loves to add other foods like kidney beans and mange tout but is less keen on the fruit. However, the basic message is the same - have fun with salads and they will keep you full, healthy and on track to be able to live well and comfortably on 2,500 or 2,000 calories a day! Lisa has now started to make herself a salad during the evening before she goes to work, to ensure she takes a healthy lunch. She found she did not have time in the morning, so simply does it the night before rather than lose out on that way of eating.

You will note I am now making positive choices to have cheese that is lower in fat and calories. It is a positive choice to eat cheese. I like cheese. The old version of me would have forced myself to give it up totally. I would have been telling myself *"Cheese is really bad for you, high in calories, and therefore you must stop it totally and forever!"*

Many other people I know do choose to give cheese up, but not me! I now understand which cheeses are better for me and I recommend you look at the various fat and calorie numbers in your App. or online to help teach you to make good food choices. I did not become a Cheese Expert overnight, I simply made sure when shopping that I paid attention to the labels on the food and slowly but surely, I worked out which versions I liked and which were the healthiest. Now I have a different question in my head.

"If there is a lower calorie version of this cheese, do you really enjoy the taste or experience of the higher calorie version enough to pay those extra calories?"

This has totally changed my outlook on what products we, as a family, choose to buy. I simply cringe when I think about how in my past life I would be asked to get some cheese on the way home and I would get the first one I saw. I know the ladies are thinking "typical man!" Yet it is true, cheese was cheese. I now see it so differently. There are some great cheeses that are low in fat, and unless I either prefer the taste of a higher calorific version or an emergency occurs and I simply have to get something very quickly (in case the Queen is popping in), I will go for the lower calorie one.

As a quick note I need to tell you this. My father-in-law, Malcolm, has a basic view of the world. If it is low calorie then it must be rubbish. Well, I am here to tell you that is simply not true. Try getting someone you trust to set up a few taste tests where you attempt to pick the low calorie version as opposed to the one packed full of calories and while sometimes you will be able to tell, it will happen far less often than you expect. Even if you start by changing your buying habits on the items where you cannot tell the difference you will have saved a whole heap of calories!

Another choice I have made is to eat less red meat. I love steak, but now I am thinner steak does not love me. It sits heavily on my stomach and I don't get the same buzz from eating it that I used to. There is nothing wrong with healthy low fat beef, but it is a once-a-month treat now rather than the three times a week base food from my past life. Once again, I do not advocate giving any food up but I promise you as you get more experienced in sticking to your daily calorie allowance you will become better at making these positive food choices.

I want to avoid going into a long list of potential food items where this positive choice can occur but, if you will forgive me, I do want to cover three others. The first is milk. I personally have skimmed milk in all my drinks because I do not really need the fat in my tea and coffee. I can cope with semi-skimmed but never have full fat. As I mentioned before, a full fat latte from my past was 250 calories a cup! I totally agree that there is nothing wrong in the slightest with a coffee in the afternoon but now I have an Americano with skimmed milk. I still have my coffee but I save 230 of the original 250 calories and without any major change in my life. Putting it bluntly, I would prefer to eat those calories on nice food rather than "waste" them on a coffee that I can still enjoy with a small change in my buying habits.

The second item to mention is alcohol. I consider myself blessed that I am a member of The Salvation Army church whose members do not drink alcohol. It has never been a temptation to me, and all those around me at work and friends know I do not drink. My delight is not a moral one, though I strongly believe that a significant amount of the hardship I see in the world is not helped by drink or the excessive use or abuse of alcohol. My delight is that I do not have to budget any calories for alcoholic drinks in my daily and weekly calorie count. The 2,500 or 2,000 daily count includes all drinks - coffees, soft drinks, beers, wines and anything else you wish to drink! In my early days I forgot that. Make sure, when you are writing your food diary, you do include ALL the calories from drinks as it will amaze you how many calories you use in this way. You recognize my normal theme and you will never hear me say stop, but just make sure you are happy you have spent your lovely calories wisely!

My last food is yoghurt. I never really ate it before I started this weight loss programme and lifestyle but now it is my first thought. I always have it as one of my courses for breakfast. The old advice to not miss breakfast has worked brilliantly for me. *I now eat MORE for breakfast than when I started to lose weight.* Yes you did read that correctly, I now eat more for breakfast than I did before. In past times, I would have started a diet and reduced my breakfast down to just a piece of toast or just a bowl of cereal. Yet now having given up giving up, my typical breakfast is as follows:

Coffee with skimmed milk
All Bran cereal (50g) with skimmed milk
Low fat yoghurt (Muller low fat) mixed up with Rice Krispies (10g)
"Crustless" toast with Flora spread and Marmite.

By shopping around on my brands I have found a variety of bread that is only 49 calories a slice and, more importantly, is NOT diet bread. It actually has no crusts but comparing that to my old bread of 120 calories a slice it is a great investment of my calories.

My new, larger, breakfast measures around 450 calories and I'm left full up. As a result I do not feel the need to snack on the train into London or to snack in the kitchen if I am working from home. It will easily get me to lunchtime at 12 noon without further food.

So in closing this chapter I would ask you to think of a few things:

- Do you have a breakfast that gets you to lunch without snacks or leaves you lacking energy?
- What foods could you change right now and replace with a lower calorie version without making any noticeable difference to your day or enjoyment of the food?
- How could you make salad a more regular part of your food regime and what would your perfect salad have in it?
- If you took your food diary and looked at it honestly, how many days in a week do you think you could add a salad at lunch or dinner time and how many calories do you think it would save you?
- How many calories do you want to use each day on drink? As a tip, work out a weekly number and divide by 7 rather than focusing on a daily number.

Chapter Eleven
Being Intentional

If any word has dominated my thinking since I seriously decided to act on my desire to lose weight it has to be the word **intentional.** Nothing positive in life happens by accident. Lottery wins start with someone buying a ticket and deciding to enter. A young couple who crash their cars into each other in a road accident and then fall in love still have to decide to ask the other one for a date rather than a court case!

Are you a victim or a player?
The older I get the more I sense in life that I have a choice to be a Victim or a Player. Victims are very easy to spot. They blame everything and everyone but themselves. This applies to every aspect of life. A bad marriage, a dislike of their job, nothing ever goes right for them, everyone else is lucky. Things go wrong and they look outside of themselves rather than how they could have made things better. If a marriage is bad, talk about it, try new things and work at it together. Give and be open. If you hate your job, go get one you DO like. Unless, of course, you would hate all jobs! Nothing goes right for me, I hear you cry! Then start to plan your life more effectively and work out what you need to do to make things go right.

As the former World Snooker Champion, Steve Davis (no relation!) used to say, "The harder I practice, the luckier I get!"

Someone who is a Player in their own life has a totally different mindset. This type of person understands that life is a precious gift and not a rehearsal. We get one attempt, so make the best of it! They make decisions and take control of things. Victims live in fear, Players live in excitement.

I always say to friends that there are four states in being a Player in life and I wanted to share my 'levels' with you.

Level One
I reached this when I worked out life was a game and I needed to embrace having as positive an experience in every aspect of my life as I could. At my wedding to Lisa we

chose a song "Life is great, so sing about it" and I stand fully by that sentiment. Life is indeed great.

Level Two

This was reached when I worked out that if life was a game it must have rules. All of the best games have rules to ensure fair play. The tricky bit about this level is I had no idea what the rules were or how to find out what they were. When it came to weight, I knew I wanted to lose pounds but really had no knowledge of how to do it, or frankly how to start. I could see there were people who succeeded with weight loss, so I knew the rules already existed, I just did not know them yet! A Victim would then say "that's not fair" but the Player intentionally says "I don't know them yet, but I am going to find out!"

Level Three

This is a fun level because when you reach this point you know what the rules are, you just are not very good at the game. My sense is lots of dieters get to this point and understand how to lose weight, but when it gets tricky they fall away. Understanding how to set the game up for success is really important and by reading this book you will be formulating ideas of how to keep self-motivated, or have others keep you motivated. The Victim will quit and will say "that's not fair, I can't do it". The Player will know that, like all games, sports or activities, it takes practice and commitment to win. I am sure we all would have liked to have been naturally able to drive a car without lessons, or to know how to use the latest technology without reading the instructions. Well, sorry, but that is not real life. Yet when it comes to weight loss, sustained weight loss, 90% of dieters will not even try to learn where the risks and dangers might be. I am thrilled you are in the 10% who do!

Level Four

This is the best level to achieve as by now you know there is a game, you know the rules, you have practiced and you're pretty good at it. This level, in weight loss terms, has to come from understanding that diets will NOT lead you to long term weight loss. Behavioural change WILL do that. It is a subtle change in mindset, but it makes a huge difference. When you understand, just as I had to understand, that if you have a healthy lifestyle, and make long term changes to your life which include watching how and what you eat, you will succeed. Holding on to a vague hope about getting smaller, that involves following a prescribed plan where you make no decisions and take no personal responsibility in becoming thinner, will actually only lead to the weight piling back on! It is not the system of weight loss that matters, it is YOU.

This advice is true in every aspect of my life. The four levels of the game are things I have seen in so many areas. It is in my heart to help as many people understand this as I possibly can. Weight is a significant issue, but it is only one of the many issues our society is facing. If we took the problem of rising divorce rates and applied the same logic it would work.

Level One would be "I hate this marriage and want out". Level Two would see the couple both understand that some people make life time commitments and marriages can work, but they have no idea how that is possible. Level Three would see that self-same couple reading books, talking to others and working out the ways that other people have cracked the same problem. Finally when they had worked out the rules of the relationship and each other's needs they have reached Level Four and have a much better chance to make things better.
I will not go into further examples but if you are struggling with any issue in your life you might find this a helpful framework.

Positive decisions

By now you may be a bit fed up of hearing this but it's important. This whole programme is based around positive thoughts and creating positive environments. One concern I have for the world is the increasing sense of entitlement that pervades. I was raised with the maxim that the world owes us nothing and I still believe all things of value need work, effort and commitment. Through the first ten chapters we have seen many examples of intentional, positive decision making. I want to go through a few with you and for the first time in the book focus more on you and your needs rather than my personal journey.

Starting the first step

Every journey has a first step. I drive a great deal and so usually my trips involve a clear destination. It is time to make a decision.

- Is weight loss important to you? Yes or No are the only options. Anything but a positive Yes is a No.
- Do you want a life where weight is no longer an issue in your life? This too is a Yes or a No. Anything but a positive Yes is a No.
- Can you write a series of reasons why losing weight is important to you? If so, please do it!
- Are you prepared to just do it and follow the advice and not spend all day questioning? Apologies but again, it is a Yes or a No.

Starting to take control

These next decisions will help you positively own success.

- Who is responsible for what you eat? Ask this question whilst standing in front of a mirror and looking forward. That will give you a clue!
- Are you committed enough to get the scales for the bathroom and kitchen and the App? The cost is around £20.00 for all of the weighing equipment in most major supermarkets. I promise you will save far more than that in weeks to come from a lower food bill.
- Are you prepared to write down what you eat for one whole week without changing your habits? You need to see the size of the problem.
- Are you prepared to stop cheating? This is another Yes or No question...sorry!
- Are you prepared to write down your starting weight and measurements and take the "pictures"?

If the answer to all these questions is "Yes" then we are in business, so you just need to do it.

Starting to shrink

Let's remind ourselves of some of the key decisions around food needed in order to lose weight on this programme.

- Can you learn to trust the calorie numbers in an App?
- Can you weigh as much of your food as possible, and enter the correct number?
- Can you plan your food for each day and then eat only that?
- Can you promise to include treats in your food intake at least once a week?
- Can you only eat food you love?
- Can you ask friends and family for help?
- Can you actively work out the times and places you will find it hard and write down a plan to make life easier at those times?
- Can you work out the overall plan for your weight loss? The start, the milestones along the way and the date by which you want to succeed?

If you can honestly say "Yes" to these questions you will succeed in all your weight objectives. If you have a few areas with which you are struggling then I would recommend looking at your motivations, and asking yourself what it is that would motivate you to change the way you are.

By now, I hope that you have the confidence to KNOW that you have the strength to lose weight by following the tips included in this book.

The following chapters will give you further help in staying safe on the quest and should help you avoid making some of the mistakes I made.

Chapter Twelve
Small Things Count

If sport can teach us anything about life, it has to be that making small improvements can have dramatic effects on the results. I always remember the dominance that Tiger Woods brought to golf. Yet, even during the hugely successful part of his career, he only averaged about 1.5 shots per round better than a mid-range professional. There was less than a 3% difference in his scores but a whole world apart in performance. Formula One motoring racing teams chase hundredths of seconds, tennis players constantly want to improve their first service percentages. Small improvements matter!

Earlier, I mentioned that this can be a long journey and it always starts with a small first step. I discovered a whole heap of small steps which I wanted to share with you as I feel they add richness to the strides you can take and may help you increase your chances of success in the same way they massively helped me.

Do not be fooled, whilst they may not take a long time to explain, these steps are really important and helpful.

Portion sizes
If you weigh your food correctly this will eventually start to become less of an issue and you will naturally find you are able to serve yourself the correct amount of food. However, here are a few practical tips that might help.

- Remember, when you eat the new sized portion you will be eating the CORRECTLY sized portion. It may look small, but the reality is that before you started this new regime you were **over eating**. Don't look at it negatively. This is a positive step, not one that takes anything away from you. You are just rebalancing to the correct healthy level of eating.
- Lord Alan Sugar always talked about how he eats with a teaspoon. I did and still do exactly the same thing. For breakfast and dessert I always use a teaspoon. This achieves two things. First, it helps me eat more slowly, and second it means I have not bolted my food down with three spoonfuls. I find this slower eating makes me feel less hungry. I always remember that it takes twenty minutes for

my brain to catch up with my stomach so it'll be a while before I realise that it is full. That's the danger zone where I can eat more than I need. By eating slowly I ensure I never feel bloated. When I eat slowly I start to gradually feel full. I can hear my body when it's warning me that I have had enough. The same will apply to you.

- Eating is a very visual activity. Think about how much detail top chefs put into the way the food is displayed on the plate. There is a close linkage to how full you feel and the size of the plate. Therefore, eat from smaller plates and your eyes will be very helpful in telling you that when you are nearing the end of the plate you are getting full.

- Have a small cereal bowl in the morning for exactly the same reasons!

- Be **intentional** when you eat. Make meals special. Sit at a table not on the couch in front of the TV. Try to eat in a deliberate way and to enjoy each and every mouthful. When I was losing weight, I was always so careful to make sure that when I ate, I noticed what I ate rather than just gobbling up food and trying to remember if I had eaten. I've also read another tip – put the fork, knife or spoon down on the table between mouthfuls and that will slow down the eating process as you concentrate on chewing what is in your mouth and savouring the flavours and textures. Whatever it takes, slow down your eating

- In every meal try to eat some of your "superfoods", your real favourites maybe which are bulky so they fill you up and are foods that make you look forward to eating. Remember, this is an eating plan for life.

- Drinking water or low sugar squash at meal times will help your system feel full. Use these special drinks as ways to naturally take on board lots of water whilst helping control any overeating.

- The body is mainly made up of water and needs lots of water to function well and effectively. Be intentional in drinking more than you currently do. When I started out I did not really like plain water all that much but whilst losing weight I was drinking over 2 litres of water every single day!

- Try to encourage the cook to keep the serving plates with the "second helpings" in the kitchen and NOT on the table. Avoid being tempted to eat something more than you intentionally set out to eat.

- Try one new food each week. If you like it, keep it on your menu but if you don't like it, at least you tried. I really had a short list of food that I ate and liked, but I kept adding items and being experimental and now I enjoy so many more food types. Foods that I may have disliked as a child are now favourites. My tastes have obviously changed but it was an intentional decision to try stuff I thought I didn't like - melon and yoghurt being my perfect examples.

How often to weigh?

I love the whole debate about weighing because, as I've said before, it just seems so simple. I personally weigh every day I can with my own scales. I do not weigh when I am travelling because I may not be able to trust the scales there and often in hotels, scales are not provided. I am so comfortable now with the programme that I personally do not need to weigh to be confident of doing the right things, so long as I am accurately entering my calorie information into my mobile App.

I have gone one step further, though, and have purchased a small set of jewellery scales which are portable and fit into my pocket when I'm travelling. I do not hesitate to weigh out my correct number of grams on to a plate when away from home. I even do this in restaurants - I will not let anything get in the way of staying healthy. I often work in the USA and portion sizes are huge. If I did not weigh my 100grams of fries I would eat about 400grams, as that appears to be the normal portion size in the States. That alone can save me from at least an extra 750 calories per day!

I know what you are thinking - he is really sad. However the reality is I will not outsource the decisions on how much I eat even to a talented kitchen worker in the US. I am now "intentional" about what I eat when I eat out in hotels!

The 2lb Rule

I have always had a problem when I started to put a little bit of weight back on. This is how it went for me. I would go out, eat a big meal as a treat and although it left me feeling bad, I soon forgot. A few more episodes like that and I might have regained several pounds. Very soon, it was half a stone and I was on that slippery slope and my belt was in need of being loosened a little again. In the past, this fear stopped me from ever enjoying such meals, which in turn meant that diets were temporary and in time meant I always put more weight back on.

This time I operated, and still do operate, to a different rule - the 2lb rule. Even if I go out and have a great meal, my weight (and yours) should not go up by more than 2lbs. Research has shown that if I have a "good day" the very next day afterwards, the fat is still in my bloodstream and not stored as body fat. It takes a couple of days for the body to convert to that lovely state! Therefore, I operate on a very tight band of my ideal weight plus 2lbs. If I am target plus 1lb I don't care, target plus 1.8lbs I also do not care. However, the second I am target plus 2lbs, I have a day or so on salad type meals to keep me at my target weight. The benefits are many; as it:

- Frees me up to enjoy any type of food!
- Allows me to make decisions on facts rather than a guess of how my weekly food intake is going. The numbers do not lie.
- Makes it easier to lose the small amount of weight without drama.
- Gives me the confidence to know I am in control.
- Means I only have to lose 70lbs once in my life! The first and the last are critical to me. Knowing I have a process that allows me to eat cake, crisps, chocolate or chips and stay focused on the early warning system allows me total freedom to be in control of my weight. I am not falling off the wagon but I am merely eating to a managed plan. There's a very big difference. I don't know about you, but the more I am forbidden something, the more I want it! I was trying to work out how much weight I had lost in my lifetime, and I stopped when I decided I had lost more than my entire body weight! If this has taught me anything it is that I want to eat more not less. The best way of eating more is to not have to diet, so I stay healthy and happy and eat what I both need and love.

How many meals do I eat?
Mentally I go into everyday with this type of plan. I eat breakfast and use approximately 500 calories of my 2,500 allowance. I do not tend to have a snack because I eat breakfast cereals that are slow to release energy and get me through to lunch. Skimmed milk and lots of water mean I use most the calories on food not drink. Lunch is usually my main meal when I tend to give myself 1,100 calories. You can eat a fair amount for 1,100 calories and once again, by using skimmed milk and water it is mainly food focused rather than drink focused.

I do tend to have a 150 calories snack mid-afternoon to keep me going up to teatime, or to get through the commute home from London. This could be fruit or chocolate, plus a coffee. Fruit is better, but I love chocolate! For tea or dinner, as some people refer to that meal, I eat about 700 calories. I have found this gives me enough calories for a coffee just before I go to bed. It is a high level plan that works for me. If I need to swap it around and eat my main meal at night that is fine but I never vary too far from this approach. If I am away and need an extra snack I make sure I take it out of the allowance for either one or both of the other main meals to balance things out.

Never go hungry
I have disciplined myself to be led by my stomach! As such, I never wait to get totally starving hungry before I eat. If I need a small snack to get to my meal I take it. I

found it counterproductive to eat when really hungry as it just made me want to eat more. Many people recommend 6 meals or snacks in a day. I use 5 but the logic is very sound.

Remembering the past
I was chatting with a shop assistant about losing weight and she had lost 6 stone or 84lbs. She said something to me I have never forgotten. I quote from my unknown friend!

"Looking back at when I was so large, I wish I knew then what I know now about healthy eating. I wish I could have had one single day in my new life to have shown myself just how wonderful life is, to have encouraged me to make the effort to take control.   Now I am thinner I so wish I could have one single day as my larger self, to clearly remember why I never want to go back!"

She was 16, and I have not edited her words at all as she floored me with the simple clarity of her thought.

Chapter Thirteen
Fit Part Two

Our first chapter on exercise was very much focused on where I started from – not exercising at all and then beginning to enjoy basic exercise. I now want to share with you the full range of exercising that I now enjoy, my reasons for intentionally working the way I do and advice on some resources that might help you. Please remember these are the exercises I enjoy and I undertake, this is not a recommendation that everyone will enjoy the same.

From the very beginning I have been aware of the body type I was looking to achieve. 'Martial Arts Expert' versus 'Body Builder' was how I processed it in my head. I was always far more focused on the 'strong but slight' look rather than a big muscled look with enormous shoulders and so my exercise reflects that desire. This is one of the reasons I recommend you know what you are trying to achieve from a looks point of view as you will undertake very different activities. As for the girls I will mention some of Lisa's routine as we go along. Both of us set out with different goals and so undertake different exercises to meet them!

Ask questions!
Being a member at my gym meant I could ask questions of people who knew more about exercise than I do. As I stated earlier I had become focused not just on weight but also by my trouser size. I was destined to be a 32 inch waist again! I spoke to about 6 people and they all said the same thing, "if you want to be thin you have to run!" I hate running! If there was a word stronger than hatred of running then that would be a better word. I really hate it!

So here I am being happy with my swimming and my rowing and riding and all of a sudden I am being told to add running. Even after getting slightly fitter I could not run for long. It goes back to my fear of failure and many bad experiences involving running at school. However, I remembered my own advice regarding trying new foods and was reminded that my adult tastes in food had changed, so hoped the same was true for exercise! When I last was running, I did not have an underlying level of fitness developing and so when I got on the treadmill, I was surprised to find it was not as bad as I had feared. I did not like it but certainly I grew not to loathe it.

A friend at the gym told me to put 0.5 degree of incline on the treadmill to make it easier. That sounded madness. How could a slope make it easier? I am glad to report that in fact the advice was correct and my heels and knees are still grateful. I just tried and did not argue too much. I then experienced a breakthrough day. I was running and saw I had just run 600 metres without stopping and it took me back to school. I have never run a whole lap of a track without stopping for a short rest. Here I was, 30 years later, having done a lap and a half and still going. So I kept going, 800 metres, 1,000 metres and finally 1,500 metres before I stopped to walk. I was amazed. I could run! Now there was no stopping me. In fact I have now set an ambition to complete a triathlon. I will not be up to the Brownlee brother's standards of Olympic Triathlon glory but I can ride and swim and run and it is there to be done! I am now working a proper running plan that is widely available on the web as a way to learn to run for 30 minutes without stopping. It involves running and walking and gradually increasing the running and reducing the walking. All based on numbers as usual and good fun!

As I say, I don't think Alistair and Jonny Brownlee are in danger of losing their gold and bronze Olympic medals, but at some point you'll see me swimming, cycling and running for my life and hopefully doing myself proud.

Lisa runs! She runs very well in fact and is far better at it than I am. Running for the girls is a great way of keeping the hips, thighs and buttocks in trim. So for all you women who have concerns in one of those areas in particular I would recommend you speak to someone about learning to run. The difference to Lisa's overall fitness has been massive and she religiously takes her music to listen to as she is on the treadmill.

Weights
When I first went to the gym I could not help but notice all these funny machines. People in agony pulling this and pushing that and I really wondered why they were doing it. I would love to say I have changed but sadly, I cannot lie. I am still baffled. I can push a fair degree of weight with my feet and legs but when it comes to lots of repetitions or "reps" as those of you 'in the know' call them, I just get bored.

Lisa uses the machines far more than I do. In particular there are machines that work both the inner and outer thigh muscles and she has found these good for helping tone her thighs even more. She started with a small number on each leg and has increased both the number and the weight she uses to get fitter in this area of her body. Whilst I do not like weights I did see a funny device with straps and lots of pretty girls using it and that looked a whole lot more fun!

TRX

If you want to really properly understand the detail about TRX systems you need to go and look it up on the internet. Needless to say I love it. Basically, it is two very strong yellow webbing straps attached either to the wall or to an overhead bar. You then use the straps to support your own body weight rather than use lots of weights. It's 'Suspension Training' and it was designed by the US Navy Seals as a way of training in the field when you did not have a gymnasium. The basic idea is that if you keep your body tight it will develop your core muscles and this makes you thinner, fitter and stronger down the central core of your body. Imagine me, standing there, with all the pretty women, leaning back on my straps pulling myself up and lowering myself down but keeping my body and legs straight and firm. It was exhausting, but I knew I had found an exercise I loved. I would stress the pretty women were just a perk and not a requirement!

I really want to recommend it to people who are losing weight because with TRX you have huge flexibility in how hard you make each lift and it builds deep strength inside you rather than muscles on your arms! As I said I didn't want to become Mr. Muscles from Maidstone! When I wanted to learn more about techniques I simply asked at the gym or went on "YouTube" for one of the hundreds of brilliant teaching videos. This was perfect for me.

Pull-ups, chin-ups and press-ups

Now I had started to enjoy more advanced levels of TRX I wanted to push the boundaries. I had never been very good at push-ups and wanted to improve. As my 'core', those muscles down the centre of my body including my stomach, back and chest, had got stronger I started to do the odd push-up at home and eventually could do ten without dying. I was proud. So proud I decided to look at the British Army Website to see how many I needed to be able to achieve to join the Army. Pure theory I promise, as I am far too old for military service. I was surprised to find out I needed to do 44 push-ups in 2 minutes. Practice was needed but in a few weeks, I finally made it. Lisa measured the number of repetitions and the children had the stopwatch. All done, I promptly collapsed in both exhaustion and delight! From none to 44 in 2minutes and it had only taken a few short months of work.

Now there was no stopping me. I had never been able to do pull-ups but the same British Army website told me I needed to be able to do 3/5 pull-ups for my theoretical military career!

At this point I must give another big "Thank You" to my friend John Cole, who is the Manager at Powerhouse Fitness, Charing Cross, in London. He is fit, seriously fit, and one of the most muscled people I know. For all of his bulk in muscle, and therefore slightly scary look, he is a lovely guy. I had tried pull-ups and I just stayed still, unmoved except for the pain on my face. John gave me two tips. Firstly, he advised I acquire a 'pull-up bar' for my doorframe. He duly went off, ordered me one and even put it up at home to help me practice. Less than £20 and I was on my way! John also told me I should look on "YouTube" at a man called "Hannibal for King". When I asked why, he smiled his wicked grin and told me to go look and I would know why! Well I tell you, I have never been so amazed in my life. Hannibal is a guy in the USA who does pull-ups, push-ups and dips on children's playground equipment. He has a cult following and now I am part of it! I am not going to try to explain just how strong Hannibal has become but he has put a whole series of demonstration and teaching videos on "YouTube". It truly is inspirational what he can make the human body do so naturally. When I thought about it I had known it all along. I watched the male gymnasts at the Olympics on the television from the comfort of my couch, and how they use the rings. It requires amazing strength. But Hannibal is different. He is simply inspiring a generation with what is possible, encouraging the world as well and after watching him I wanted to be able to do it. I set a goal of being able to complete 25 pull-ups (palms facing away from me on the bar) and 25 chins-ups (palms facing towards me on the bar), as well as 25 with my hands at 90 degrees to those positions. The chins-ups work my arm muscles and the pull-ups work my back and shoulder muscles. The other exercise works both muscle groups but they share the work. So whilst I doubt Hannibal will ever read this book, I truly want to say "Thank You" to him for showing me what I could achieve! Please watch the videos.

I went back to my Apps. again and discovered a pull-up plan to help me get there and I was away. At the time of writing I can manage the required number of chin-ups and nearly 20 of the pull-ups. All in all, not bad for a guy who could not run 400 metres!

Core strength – The benefits - size and skin reduction
While I was watching Hannibal's amazing videos I found another giving a 100 second core strength routine. I liked this idea because while I could always find good reasons not to go to a gym, it was impossible not to find 100 seconds in a day to do an exercise routine. Think about it – 100 seconds is not even 2 minutes. It was about me identifying another risk to my future and developing a plan to mitigate it and make this plan work, rather than allowing any victim-like behaviour to develop. The 100 second core strength routine involves 5 sections of 20 seconds each.

- 20 seconds on my back with feet 6 inches off the ground remaining still.
- 20 seconds in the same position but kicking my feet like I was swimming back stroke, alternating each foot.
- 20 seconds moving my legs from horizontal to vertical (flat to straight up) while ensuring my feet stayed locked together. When doing this your legs should go from flat to 90 degrees upwards.
- 20 seconds doing ab-crunches / sit-ups.
- Finally, after turning over on to my front, 20 seconds performing a plank holding my body tight and straight resting on my toes and elbows. This means that only your toes and elbows should be touching the floor and your whole body is rigid, like a plank! It's a tough routine but after a few weeks it really started tightening up my muscles and I was really getting trimmer. This exercise definitely helped me reach my 32 inch waist target. However, the exercise routine has also helped me shrink my skin. When you lose a lot of weight excess skin is a real issue. However, even in this area I have made huge progress and commend exercise as a great way of improving a tough situation.

Cross Core 180
Having loved TRX, John called me very excitedly to tell me about a new type of device that was being used in the US military called Cross Core 180. Once again, I will not spend time explaining it in detail as it is very similar to the TRX, yet very different. However, the system/equipment is easier to take travelling with you and I now have one set up at home to help me work out when I cannot get to the gym. You can set it up at home by attaching it to any horizontal bar or wall mounted bracket you may have. We have one bedroom with a rafter across the top of the ceiling and I have hung my Cross Core from the ceiling so I can exercise to my heart's content.
I wanted to end this chapter focusing on what I have learned so I can help you. On the exercise front, I knew nothing really about anything which I needed to do to get fitter. People willingly helped me. Undoubtedly, I am fitter today than at any point in my life and happy that it has helped me stay focused on my vision of what I wanted to look like. Exercise helps me be able to eat more, it helps keep my body burning energy effectively and it reduces the effects of stress. Thanks to all those people who encouraged me to not give up on exercise!

Exercise is a very personal activity. I have explained some routines that work for the men. Lisa uses running, weights, swimming and riding the exercise bike together with the odd aerobics class to manage her exercise requirements. However, the main message here for both men and women is this. Know what you are aiming for in terms of body type and talk to someone at the gym about specific exercises that are good to meet your goals. Women in particular are sensitive to certain bits of their body that they focus on. For some it is thighs, others hips, and for some others it is stomach shape or general size. Make sure you understand what you want to achieve and I guarantee you that you will find a fun, successful series of exercises that you will both learn to enjoy and that will support your weight loss goals.

Chapter Fourteen
Clothing

Having made so much progress on how to lose weight we can now focus on three chapters of pure unadulterated fun! For me, there seemed little point to all the hard work if I was not allowed some fun.

My old wardrobe

I am certain that what I am about to describe is very common among the people reading this book. I know so many people who feel the same, and have had the identical experience. You see, I did not seem to ever have enough wardrobes. It didn't matter how many I bought it was never enough. This was for one reason and one reason alone. You see I kept all my clothes! I had more clothes than most department stores.

Let's start with trousers. A long time ago I had been a 36 inch waist and I had trousers that fitted me. Then, sadly, I expanded and had to buy 38 inch trousers to fit better and more comfortably. However, what originally started as "just one pair" turned into more and more, as the length of time as a 38 inch waist increased. In time, I had as many 38 inch trousers as I did 36 inch pairs. Yet I simply could not throw them away. It would have meant admitting to me, let alone Lisa, that I was bigger than before and had no hope of returning to my smaller size. There was always hope! So I dutifully filled up my wardrobe until I could not cope with any more trousers!

This logic was fine until I repeated the same behaviour when I went from a 38 inch waistline to 40 inches. As I confessed earlier, it was when I was on the journey from 40 inches to a size 42 that I decided enough was enough. Every time I ran out of room, I would box up the clothes and either put them in the bottom of my wardrobe or up in the attic. Of course, this applied to every item. Coats, jackets, suits, shirts, T-shirts, polo shirts and jumpers, nothing was exempt from this routine.

I know from watching Lisa that the same was true for her with dresses, skirts and all her clothing. I dread now to think just how many items of clothing we hung on to. I also noticed that when I started to sort out all these clothes, I also possessed little imagination. I had bought lots of similar items. I had many pairs of trousers of similar colours but in different sizes. I guess it was partially because I liked the style, or colour, but maybe also to disguise the fact I was going up in size. If I had added up the total cost of all these clothes I am sure I would have been shocked. What a waste of resources, both financial and material!

I have sent it all away. I kept nothing. The majority went to the recycling clothing banks and the charity shops of Medway and Maidstone, and a few select items went to eBay. They are all gone. I wanted and needed a new, fresh start when it came to clothing.

My new wardrobe
At the beginning of my weight loss programme, many of my clothes were getting tight and so my first experiences of clothes, in this new world, were that, amazingly, they started to fit again. However, as I lost more weight I soon started to get to a place where I needed some clothes that actually did fit properly. Work was an issue because I still had to look smart. Whilst I had boxes of older clothes they somehow did not feel right. My solution was to buy a smaller 38 inch size set of clothes. I had stopped being an XL and was now just a Large and enjoying that fact. However, with such a variation in the sizes of different brands it was hard to know exactly where I stood and there was an issue of on-going cost. If I was going to drop pounds as I planned, then I would need clothes that fitted, but that could end up draining my bank account. I'd be thin but broke. I am really glad I bought good but cheaper clothes as I lost weight. The supermarkets were indeed super! I was in smaller clothes and not investing a fortune. Deep down, I hoped these clothes would not be required for very long so they didn't have to last forever.

This was the way I progressed as I got smaller. I bought the smallest wardrobe of cheaper clothes I could find and worked from that limited base but always ensuring I wore clothes that fitted. I now felt better in the smaller size of clothes. Like many larger people, I had always preferred the baggy look but as I got trimmer I wanted to feel clothes against my skin. There was another benefit of the new wardrobe - disposing of the larger clothes somehow made the past disappear more quickly. If you throw away the clothes that are too big, there is nowhere to hide if you slip and start to increase your weight. A perfect motivation for me! I could not have gained weight otherwise I risked having to go naked! Not a pretty sight!

In time, as I moved from 38 inches to 36 inches, I decided I was getting nearer the end of the journey and so I bought a pair of nicer mid-price jeans. The three months they fitted went very fast and in fact I only wore them a few times, but I have never felt as good as the day I passed them on to a friend. This is a key mental point on the weight loss journey. I had learned a new behaviour for disposing of clothes I would not need again. I was not going to regain the lost pounds, and I wanted the discipline of knowing that life would start to get expensive if I did. Once I got to a 34 inch waist measurement, I started to see very significant sales in the shops. Everywhere I looked stores seemed to be offering 50, 60 and even 70% discounts. It was at this point I decided I could start to buy more 'long term' clothes and began to realise that some of the designers I had heard about but never worn, actually made quite nice clothes that fitted me. I still buy basic items from supermarkets and the high street as I can't see the point of paying more than I need to but in addition, I have embraced the new concept that nice clothes make me feel special.

The larger clothes I used to wear are now replaced with clothes that show my shape. I feel confident in my appearance. Not arrogant, but confident and I think after all these years I am worth the odd great item of clothing in a sale.

New clothes made me feel more professional

Whenever I see clothes which I know will look great on Lisa, I really struggle with temptation to buy them for her, far more than if they were for me. She is now down to her final size and wears a UK size 8/10 in most items. She is smaller than the day we were married in 1993 and before the two children, and is just simply perfect in my eyes. I can confess to you, but you mustn't tell her (it is a secret!), that she is no more perfect in my eyes as size 8 then when she was a 12 or 14 but I now see in her eyes a new level of contentment. She is in a place where she feels she is the best size for her. This is the difference. In the same way I am more content in my new size, so is Lisa. Contentment is infectious! She is balanced in what she buys but keen to look her best. Lisa is a great example to me and our children and is proof that the way you look affects the way you behave.

I have already mentioned Steve Davis, the former Snooker World Champion, and he used to speak about how he loved to play in his dinner shirt and bow tie. It made him act a great deal more professionally and helped his concentration. In fact, Steve was going to work and he dressed to perform! Clothing and the way I am dressed also affects the way I feel about myself. It is only my opinion, but in the casual world in which we now live, too few people seem to invest in making an effort to look smart. Looking smarter, leaner and presentable has helped me feel special again. It has re-energised me in nearly every area of my life.

It has also had many other benefits beyond how I feel within myself. Most significantly, I have had times in the past when I have been tempted to always hide myself away in sports gear, loose t-shirts and frankly not make much of an effort about my appearance. Not anymore. If I start to let those types of negative, indifferent behaviours into my life, it might spread to all the other facets of my existence as well. My time keeping has improved massively, and my desire to finish jobs around the house has increased. When Lisa leaves me lists of jobs to do, I seem to get through them faster, and in a more focused way. I make the bed every morning and don't get tempted to leave it messy. I am sure you get the picture. My new clothes have literally wrapped me in a new set of more professional behaviours, not just at work but in every area of my life. Intentional clothing has certainly lead to unintentional benefits for me, my family, friends and folk I work with.

Let's not beat around the bush, I now enjoy shopping. I love seeing nice things at great prices and every so often giving into temptation. Before the weight loss, I loved shopping and did not give in, as it made far less difference to me. One baggy shirt or another is much the same. I know it sounds vain, but I prefer the new feelings to the old. I know not everyone has the resources to splurge from time to time and I am privileged to be able to do so, but there are always ways around the issue, like the great sales that shops often offer. I wonder if you would feel the same as I do now when you at last discover the joy of shopping for clothes that not only fit but make you feel GOOD.

Chapter Fifteen
Travel and Holidays

In earlier chapters I have mentioned the need to be intentional around managing my own high risk areas. Over the next few chapters I will be talking through a couple of those that existed for me. They were very real then and they are still real today. I love to travel. My job means that I travel the world and so far I have worked in 38 different countries. I am convinced that part of my problem with my weight has been the 'dangers' of food and travel. So I knew I needed a plan to mitigate risks relating to whenever I travel. My two normal reasons for travelling are work and holidays with the family. So I prepared my thoughts to ensure I could undertake these two activities that were, and still are, very important aspects of my life.

Beware of travelling for work!

As a Project Manager I have noticed that the world is shrinking but even though modern technologies are advancing, the need for face-to-face interaction still very much exists. When I travel the main food/overeating risks that occur can be identified in three areas. Firstly, the journey itself can be very tricky. Secondly, living in hotels and eating hotel food always carries a risk of a high calorie lifestyle and lastly, entertaining when away.

Is the journey essential?

As I've said, my work means that I travel a great deal, so without a doubt the first action I needed to take was to avoid travelling unless it was essential to the success of the work project. This is a good plan on so many levels.

From a cost perspective it is good stewardship of the company's finances to only travel when needed. As most of my journeys involve intercontinental flying, I am permitted to fly in Business Class and as we all know this is not cheap!

Related to this is the environmental benefit of the reduced numbers of planes flying around, and also the reduced weight of the plane, which affects the CO_2 emissions of the flight. As we all know reducing CO_2 emissions is a good plan! However, the two main benefits for me of a reduced commitment to travelling are the avoidance of time away from the family and the ability to stay in my normal regulated food regime.

I promise you, travelling for work is not at all glamorous. For the first few trips it is exciting but after a while I genuinely lost any excitement in flying. So much so, that now I can be asleep before the plane has taxied from the stand and fail to notice the plane take off.

The ability to avoid all three of the risk areas is a massive up side to using one of the many virtual working tools. Telephone, communicator, Skype, video conferencing all play their part in helping to avoid travel and as such they will help me stay thinner, but taking food temptations away from me completely was the key to the travel I had to undertake.

Temptations on the day of travel
I have always found the actual day of travel to be very difficult from a food perspective. Here's an example of me travelling to the USA. I would start by getting up for my normal breakfast, then journey the 70/80 miles to Heathrow Airport where I would arrive just in time for lunch. Fresh from checking in I would sit down to lunch around 12noon. However, once the plane takes off I am then offered coffee and nuts, and a full 3-course meal. All this assumes I have missed any temptation while waiting at the airport. It could be coffee or doughnuts jumping out as just a couple of potential attractions. After a number of hours it will be time for another meal before I finally land at my destination. Also bear in mind that during this whole day I've done little but sit down – in a car or train, in the airport waiting area and in the plane. Not much exercise has been undertaken!

Sadly, my arrival in Houston, Texas is not the end of my problems. I find that I am now six hours behind London time and my body thinks it is tea time! Invariably, I start to feel hungry again and I want another main meal, before going to bed. All this means that in just one day, I could easily have several extra meals and still not feel that I have over eaten. Logically, if I have an additional meal on the way to the USA, I should require one fewer meal on the way home when I'm 'going forward' rather than 'going back' 6 hours, but it never happens like that. The truth is, in my experience, travelling adds meals to your day. It is tiring and puts you in places where it is really easy to snack on "rubbish" food.

Under my programme of risk mitigation this is what I now do to avoid any problems. I still have breakfast as normal with the customary 450 calories. After I check in at the airport, I go and have a proper healthy meal. Usually this would involve a green salad and chicken, together with a light dessert. After takeoff, when the nuts or snacks

---

are offered I keep them for later in the flight and do NOT have the meal offered to me on the plane. If I feel in need of a small snack I eat the snacks I've stowed away earlier, and drink lots of water. When the second/tea-time meal comes I have just a sandwich which allows me to enjoy a light additional meal that evening in Houston, and only be slightly over my calories for the day. This is a very intentional plan. I set out, knowing I will eat too much on that one day, but knowing it would have been much worse if I had not planned my food intake in advance. I do this journey from London to Houston so often now that I can put the food into my App. before I start the day and then I am just delivering to the plan. In the past over the course of the travel days, I would eat around 5,000 calories but now it is only 3,000 and very little damage, if any, has been done to my weight as a result. So if I have any advice for you when travelling it is - plan the day and you can cope just fine.

Hotel food – A survival guide

Where on earth do we start on managing calorie intake in hotels? The word 'hotel' has a second meaning after 'accommodation' and that is 'nightmare place to stay thin'. Breakfast is often included in the overnight charge, and the chances are I will be offered a HUGE cooked breakfast with masses of food that I would not normally eat. I have now disciplined myself to stick to 500 calories at this first meal of the day. For variety, I sometimes have bacon and egg or even a croissant but I never go for a full "eat as much as I can" type breakfast. In my old life I could have consumed a whole day's calories and still have made it to the office without any trouble at all. When travelling, I usually find it impossible to find skimmed milk, so I assume the worst and default to counting my milk input as semi-skimmed and that's what is recorded in my App. programme.

Because I am eating breakfast in a sensible way, I find getting to lunch to be surprisingly easy. I need to make sure that I do actually eat the 500 calories because if I under consume at breakfast, I then need a snack. Lunch is usually at the office and so I simply ensure I make a smart choice similar to that which I would have at home. In the US, that means focusing on the portion size, and often I will throw away or not take half of the food offered and still eat as much as my usual lunch.

Dinner back at the hotel is always a tricky situation because I never really know what I am eating. What was it cooked in? How much did it weigh? I am sure you understand why, even now, I make sure I use my travel scales if I am dining alone to get a rough idea of the portion size and calorie intake. Once again, I am intentional, to ensure I do not over eat by falling into the trap of someone in the hotel kitchen, who I have never met, deciding my weight. You will not be surprised to know that I do let myself have one meal where I have a treat of steak or something similar on each trip. In the main though, I try to stick to eating sensible foodstuffs that I know from experience are good for me. That includes lots of white meat like turkey and chicken garnished with a tasty salad. I eat fewer chips/fries and potato crisps now, but I do confess that I do still indulge a little when I'm working away. I also find that working in the USA as much as I do, I have had to get used to it being very difficult to find vegetables, or certainly plain vegetables. Potato is normally fried in some way, as are most other items but salads are widely available, as long as you remember to not have it covered in cheese!

During my time in the hotel I reference what I am eating across the whole week. It is less about an individual day, and more about making sure I am balanced over all 5 days of the trip. If I know I have a heavy food day booked on Day 3, I make sure Days 2 and 4 are more sensible. I focus on balance and not eating too much red meat and I assume I am eating on the high side of the calorie count if in any doubt. However, I really concentrate on sticking to my 2,600 calories, which is now what I need to maintain my weight. In the old days I would gain at least 3lbs on a trip to the USA but it is with some pride I can say I now work in the USA and can come home no heavier than when I left. I do not drink alcohol so I stick to low calorie drinks, as ever, but I would need to factor in wine and spirits if I was a drinker. Finally, unlike the old days I use the hotel gym a great deal now when away. I only stay in hotels where they provide a gym for the guests. At least once each day I will undertake exercise either in my room or at the gym in the hotel. In the past, I would let all exercise fall by the wayside but now I use my trips as a positive way to undertaking more physical activity. I am away from the children so I'm freed up from 'Dad's Taxi' driver duties. Yet again, exercising whilst away and using the gym is intentional so I need to make sure I pack my trainers and kit. But the exercise also keeps me feeling healthy and I think helps me cope with the inevitable jet-lag.

Entertaining when working
I use the same plan for entertaining as I do for the main meal when I am alone but there is a difference. When dining alone I will eat two courses and when in a group there is peer pressure to have three courses. Nowadays, I am happy to either have a salad as a starter or simply pass up the offer and not feel at all bad about doing so. I do not know why I never felt empowered to politely refuse, but I always found myself eating large meals when I entertained or was being entertained.

The other challenge is when you do not get to choose the restaurant. This is where experience will help. If you weigh everything at home you will develop an eye that will allow you to make a better food choice when dining in a restaurant. The best way I have found to handle this is to have an approximate calorie count in my head. I always remember what I eat and not what I am served. I try to ensure I eat similar sized meals to when at home but it is far harder in a group. I have also trained myself not to eat bread in this environment. In truth it is very hard indeed to have a "good" food day when being entertained but the plan is very much to make sure I do not go silly with my eating. As ever, I keep focused on a long term sustainable lifestyle and it is essential to be able to go out and have a nice meal. All of the discipline I have learned is required to keep me eating slowly and intentionally and drinking lots of low calorie drinks.

On a slightly humorous note, for those who know me well, I have one extra piece of advice. Talk! If you are talking you are not eating. I can imagine a few friends tempted to comment on how that explains a lot about me!

I am keen we all plan our food intake each day and use our skills from home to estimate as well as we can our portion sizes while away from home. This will make sure we do not have a very bad food day outside of our safe environment at home and come out of the travel experience having had fun but not so stuffed that we return significantly heavier. As you can tell my plan when entertaining is to minimalise the damage!

Holidays

In many ways the challenges around holidays or vacations mirror those for travelling away from home for work. During holidays we are presented with new foods, have less control of portion sizes and temptation is all around.

I will not duplicate advice and experience from the work section so my view on breakfast remains unchanged. However, the ability to self-cater and use your normal brands should not be ignored because that can help you take temptation away when you are on holiday. A breakfast cooked by someone else is always a wonderful experience and if you want to try it, that is fine, but just ensure it is no more often than once every three days and things will be OK. However, try to think of these things when you are booking the holiday and not just when you arrive.

Lisa and I have recently, when on our holidays, moved to a two meal day. As we are on holiday we get up later and then go for a bigger breakfast/lunch. This has meant that we can spread our calories in a different pattern when on vacation. Breakfast has been typically around the 1,000 calories mark and the main meal at night around the 1,500 calories level. We have encouraged each other when feeling in need of a snack to have a drink, but on those occasions when only ice cream will do, we make good choices on the specific ice cream and make sure that it is not the highest fat or highest calorie option. We enjoy our food but not without thinking about what we are doing to our calorific bank account. I know it sounds silly but now I wear tighter clothes it really helps me on holiday to feel when I am full and not to overeat. We try not to sit around getting bored which helps avoid the temptation to snack. We all know the devil finds work for idle hands and when I am on holiday if I am not busy, I want to eat! We now have activity holidays such as skiing or days full of planned adventure – rolling around on the water in inflatable giant hamster wheels and climbing trees at Centre Parcs!

Although this section is aimed at some of the practical tips I use to stay in a sensible weight range when on holiday I do want to end with this honest confession. When I go on holiday I expect to put on one or two pounds in weight per week. I do not worry about it, or even let it enter my head. I use common sense to make sure I do not put on half a stone or 7lbs but I KNOW that when I get home and return to my normal regime I will be back on plan. Although it sounds like I'm now a bit obsessive about what I eat and when, I'm not, and I still believe that holidays are for relaxing. This is a lifetime programme so you need to have fun and let your hair down on the food control once in a while.

If, before I started, you had told me that I could have had this type of control over food I would not have believed you. You will develop experience that will prove to you that you can lose a pound or two very easily when you are home. Just make sure you do not get too far off your target weight during your holiday. The simple fact is that a large number of people start to put weight on by not losing holiday excesses. So, my final word is have a great time when away but be doubly careful when you return to stick rigidly to your calorie count for that next week with no excuses. I promise it will work for you, just as it has for me.

Chapter Sixteen
Birthdays and Celebrations

Despite my best efforts I seem to have a birthday ever single year! I try so hard to defer them but to no avail. As well as my birthday, Lisa also has one as do each of the children. Our extended family is also rather large and therefore we celebrate lots of birthdays, anniversaries and other family celebrations during which will practice our eating skills. In addition there is Christmas, Easter, and Thanksgiving. In England, Sunday roast dinners are a tradition and I love my Sundays so I need to add that meal to this section, because for us to have a fun life and a fulfilling time with food we simply have to be able to enjoy these experiences.

Why do we do it?

I have asked myself so many times over the years why it was I felt the need to overeat whenever I went to one of the celebration meals. There seemed to be a correlation between my attendances at a family "do" and feeling full and bloated and generally fat the following day. I know I am not alone in this. I know so many of us experience those same feelings, so why do we do it? I am convinced that the main issue is we like our friends and family to have fun and enjoy exciting food that leaves them feeling content. We all feel temporarily happier after eating sweet and sugars. Simple carbohydrates do it every time! We enjoy that rush of sugar ourselves and because we want to make our friends and family happy, we serve food which we know will make them feel good. After all, we are not stingy, are we?

What shall we arrange for Gran?

My first question in this section touches on the organization for family events. Do they really have to involve large amounts of food? We have just had a perfect example of this with Lisa's mother celebrating her 77th birthday. We wanted to get everyone together at her house in Guernsey and so a cunning plan was hatched to ensure she was out of the house.   Laura and a few of her cousins were duly sent to take their Gran to a local tea shop to have a chat, and Operation Celebration was underway.

Historically we have put everything on a big table and served a buffet meal of mainly finger food. This would include pastry, fried food, crisps and nuts etc. My experience of this type of meal is very poor. Intentional eating is hard when so much delightfully tasting grub is put in front of me. This, added to lots of chatting which prevented me thinking about each mouthful, meant I ate far too many calories! This time around, we were really pushed for time to get things set up and Lisa prepared a few lower calorie "casserole" type dishes. A chicken dish, a sausage and bean casserole and a vegetarian quiche (with potato and no pastry) was put together. It was quicker to make, easier to serve and definitely felt far more like a meal than an extended buffet. The salad, rice and potatoes meant that every one of the 14 guests left well fed with healthy and filling food, and temptation was removed. Dessert was a fruit salad and of course we had to have a slice of birthday cake! All this occurred with a little bit of planning.

Good celebration outcomes

The conclusion of this part of the story is simple. With proper planning, celebrations can be excellent and have great calorific and enjoyment outcome. You may recall I mentioned my lovely 'Spice Girls Question' - '"Tell me what you want, what you really, really want." Good celebrating is defined by making sure you add the extra dynamic of healthy and filling food to celebration meals. Culturally we have grown up with 'party food' but who decided that this party food had to be so bad for each of us?

There is, for sure, a sweet spot of having a great celebration, enjoying eating, and not damaging our weight. It does exist but we have to consider this in our objectives for the time together. We do this when we deal with children. I see numerous parents trying really hard to get their children to eat well and avoid high fat foods and sweets, yet when we entertain adult friends and family members we seem to ignore the same responsibility for looking after our guests.

Christmas and New Year

Is it me or has the Christmas period got longer? I always remember celebration on December 24th, 25th and 26th, but now there seem to be parties on each and every day between Christmas and New Year. It feels like 10 days of forced eating when it comes to the end of year period. In addition the extra nuts, chocolates and sweets, together with mince pies and other festive goodies make this time of year very risky indeed from a weight perspective

Planning my food is never as important as it is at this time of year and I wanted to share with you some of the ways I have managed to survive this experience whilst still enjoying a super time and not adding too much to my weight. I started off with an honest assessment of my weight on the 24th December. I understand, expect and have accepted that over Christmas I will put on a small amount of weight. This time of year, and holidays, are the only time I allow myself to vary from the 2lb rule. Last Christmas, I planned to have fun up to 4lbs over my target weight.

Let me put this into some context - **an extra 4lbs of fat is equal to an extra 14,000 calories of food intake, which is not far off an extra week's worth of food!** So I did not think I was being mean with myself for this allowance. I gave myself the week from 24th December until 2nd January to use my deliberate and intentional weight increase.

Despite the Christmas and New Year excitement, I remembered to think of my food as my calorie bank account and started to look at all the food risk times over that period and prioritise which meals or moments were most important to me and which would most likely cause me trouble. In the same way as I cannot spend money twice, I was committed to not eating my calories twice. I also decided to expand my exercise routine. There was nothing to stop me targeting to exercise for at least 400 calories each day. This would mean that I had a little more flexibility with the total number of calories and it would help my body burn calories effectively.

I am sure one or two of you are thinking this is a lot of planning when you want to be having a party and in many ways you are correct. It does require discipline and commitment. But I want to take you back right now to my story. Remember, I was unable to climb in the tree ropes with my children and could not make the right memories with them? What is most important, a bit of planning or continuing to live in such a way that the plan is thrown in the bin? I really want to call it as it was. In the old days, I would have allowed myself to put on half a stone at least or maybe even more. However, last Christmas, I managed to find the discipline to eat sensibly and in a structured way. I had a brilliant festive season but I did not need to wastefully eat to enjoy myself. I found the gift of not being out of control far more enjoyable than a bag of peanuts!

Stay focused
So, these are my key tips for celebrations and as usual I end with some questions and some thoughts.

- Which is more important, all your dreams and goals or a few handfuls of fatty foods? I know that, deep inside, you know the answer.

- What is it you really, really want? Where does the desire come from that means you want to spend your food bank calories and then a whole lot more? Food eating can be totally habitual at this time of year and it does not really make the season that 'special'. The special nature of the Season of Goodwill is created by the people, the family and friends around you, and the understanding of what you are celebrating. Your dreams for a healthy you are far too important to casually throw away and risk a permanent "giving up" of your new regime and behaviours at just the time of year when we are reminded of the hope which Christmas brings to the world.

One member of our family has a brilliant story to tell. Their father was an alcoholic but was amazingly converted to a deep Christian faith and never touched a drop of alcohol again. He always said that he was not given the strength to give up the booze, but had to be given the strength to stay sober every single day for the rest of his life. Just one day at a time. It's an amazing story but one that is very relevant for us at this point. Over the time you are on the programme you will learn that success is a daily activity. If you do well on a given day and eat well, it is a great achievement and one of which you should be proud. However, tomorrow takes a new determination to repeat the same behaviour. Equally, if you have a bad day, it has gone and there is nothing you can do about it except to learn and not repeat the same mistake tomorrow. Weight loss occurs when you decide to have more good days than bad ones!

One important part of the former alcoholic's story is that he never ever went again into a public house or bar, because he was concerned that the smell of the alcohol and the atmosphere would ignite something within him. He made an intentional decision to avoid temptation. When it came to sweets, nuts and chocolates this last Christmas season, we only had a very small amount either in the house or on display. We wanted to follow the same advice and not put temptation in our line of sight. So what actually happened to my weight last Christmas? I know you want to know! Well I went up 2lbs which I had discarded before the end of the first week in January.

Success has not been about what I eat or don't eat. It has been about me understanding myself and how I react in certain situations.   I have learned to think and plan. I have learned to take control of my size by simply stepping into the space of deciding what I eat. Finally, I have learned that by understanding the risky areas and potential problem situations, and taking myself to a difference space, I have the absolute best chance of meeting my goals.

All because I listened to Mel B, Mel C, Sporty, Posh and Scary and decided what I wanted...what I really, really wanted!

Chapter Seventeen
Everything Changes

As we start to come to the end of both our journey and of this book, I want to give you some insight into what has changed in my life over the past year or so as a result of my embracing this new life. After a great deal of thought, I came to the distinct conclusion it was far easier to tell you what had stayed the same, but this journey is all about doing the RIGHT thing not necessarily taking the EASIEST route.

Husband/Partner
I now feel that I am a far more confident person, who has managed to find the true inner me. I know people who know me well will laugh when I say I have grown in confidence but it is genuinely true. Maybe they've always thought I was confident but I've always been my harshest critic and I finally feel I have proved to myself that I can control the inner me and remove the "victim" aspect from my life.

Lisa has been so supportive and I am so thrilled we succeeded on our journey together. It is another bond and part of our life where the two of us have supported each other and that makes me feel special. In finding the level of discipline that this programme has taught me, I have proved to be far more reliable at helping around the house which, as I've said before, is shown in lots of silly little things. I put things away, I load the dishwasher, and I don't wait to be asked (as much). I take pride in closing items on the family action list and a whole lot besides! I won't list everything but that list is endless. Is this due to me being thinner? In some small way maybe it is. I am fitter and stronger and so can keep going for longer. However, in the main it is the result of the behaviours that I have learned by simply accepting that I can comply, take control and be intentional.

I certainly feel a whole heap more special when I go out with my sweetheart. She deserves not a thin me, but the best me that I can be. For me and me alone, I feel that the best me looks much more like the "new" me than the "old" me.

Father/Parent
I have always been concerned that I have been setting a poor example to my children when it came to food. I wanted to cure that and I am now much happier that they are

experiencing a proper, sustainable message in my relationship with what I eat. I am sure I am not alone when I say that my children absorb my actions like sponges. I can see them changing their own behaviours and attitudes to what they choose to eat. I can see then focusing on their fitness and their wellbeing. In short, I am a much better example and Josh and Laura are responding in a positive way.

I shudder when I think about the poor example I have set these two beautiful people. They are both wonderfully generous, polite, kind and great company. They are all I could ever want as a parent. Of course, they can be noisy, loud, moody, messy and many other things, and most of these attributes they have learned directly from me! How my own parents must laugh when I moan about untidy bedrooms when I think of what mine used to be like. Now I am sure that I am a better example than I was in the past. In short, my children are seeing an intentionally better example, and I rejoice.

As a son
My own parents have been such a brilliant support to me and I wanted them to know and see I was able to be healthy long term. In fact I wanted them to get the satisfaction of seeing me conquer possibly the hardest internal struggle in my life. They have helped me by gently keeping me focused. My own father went on a significant diet at a similar age and knowing he managed to achieve his weight goals and stay at that weight into his 70s has been a huge encouragement to me.

As an employee
I have been privileged enough to work with my current employer for over a decade. The company has always been the most wonderful support to me, enabling me to undertake challenging and rewarding assignments and also in the way it encourages the staff to try to stay healthy.

In a work environment we have to work with many people on a virtual basis and it is possible for me to not see or meet colleagues for many months. I have laughed with so many friends at work when they failed to recognize me in the canteen, or while at a coffee machine. I will not try to quantify in my own words how things have changed at work but I will share a few of the comments I have been given and leave it for you to decide if these are outcomes you might desire.

- You look far more "professional"

- You come across as "more assured, more measured"
- "How on earth have managed that?"
- "Before you were a lovely kind looking guy, now you look more purposeful"
- "You look great"

I recognize all these comments and I feel more assured and able to stand my ground when I feel passionately about something. I am also delighted that I managed to make the change, and I feel great. I do not want to end this section without a final word to all readers who manage people. I had a line manager, who I count as a mentor and friend, who in several reviews and development meetings took a risk and commented on my weight. He told me I would cope better with stress if I lost a few pounds. He told me I would cope more with all the travel if I was lighter. In short, he took a risk that I would not get all upset and sensitive but that I would take his comments in a positive way to deliver more to the company and myself. I recognized that he cared, not just about what I did for the company, but for the "whole" me. He gave me encouragement to use the health and fitness centre that we are blessed to have in the basement at work, and taught me to take time to exercise to ensure "peak" performance. How many leaders take that risk? How many leaders bother that much, to step out and care in a genuine and authentic way? I quoted earlier one of my favourite sayings - *"I can't hear what you are saying because your actions are speaking so loudly"* - well in this case I heard the words and my line manager's actions spoke volumes.

Many other hats
Like everyone else I wear many hats in life. At the badminton club, I run faster, try harder, play longer and am a better partner since I got fitter. As a soprano cornet player in a Salvation Army band, I can play higher and louder than ever before now that I have such a strong core set of muscles. I wish I had found that out 25 years ago! Better late than never!

As a member of the school "mums" I am not as late as I used to be and the others don't have to call me on the days I am due to collect my daughter to say "are you picking Laura up?"

As a commuter I am nicer to sit next to as I fit on just one seat, not one and half.

It all boils down to one thing - as a man I have found peace. In losing weight, I achieved something special. In the USA, people have been simply brilliant. So many people have said "well done, you must be so delighted" or made other comments which include some form of "congratulations". It seems far more culturally acceptable to articulate those messages of congratulations in the USA than on the British side of the 'Pond'.

I believe every person has a duty to strive to grow. Each person should continue to learn more and become experienced in different areas of their life. However, it does not stop there. We all have a duty to give and to help others reach their full potential in equal measure to that which we have been given. I have been given so much and I now have to complete that task by trying to give encouragement and knowledge to others. As a personal reflection, we all have many battles we have to fight in our lives. At least in this one, I take confidence that I came out on top!

Chapter Eighteen
Final Reflections

	Start	Finish
Age:	44	45
Gender:	Male	Male
Height:	6ft 0 in	6ft 0 in
Starting Weight:	249lbs	178lbs
Waist Size:	42 in	32 in
Chest Size:	48 in	40 in
Hip Size:	48 in	38 in
BMI:	33.80	24.1
Clinical definition:	Obese	Normal
Target Weight:	178lbs	Achieved
Target loss:	71lbs	Achieved

I have reprinted above the chart I shared earlier but this time I have included my end numbers. I hope you find them interesting.

I set out to explain what happened and I hope while reading this book you have smiled at some of the crazy things that have occurred. I also hope that you have been challenged to think about your weight loss in a new way.

Most of all, I hope you have been encouraged to believe that this story, the story of an ordinary man, could truly be your own story. Man or a woman, it does not matter...it could be you!

I have tried to keep the narrative in the first person and wherever possible not to lecture others but rather to just reflect my thoughts as they applied to me. If at any point I have offended anyone, please accept my apologies right now, as that was most surely not my intention. To all my American friends, I apologise for using far too many "U"s in my English words!

I have tried to set out the questions at the end of some of the chapters to help you follow some sort of process but it is worth re-visiting the top 25 steps I believe you need to think about to start you on your journey to the YOU that you have always dreamed about.

In an attempt to keep costs down I have not shared pictures in the book. This is intentional too but I will be putting many photographs of "before and after" on the website.

Please find these at:
www.finallyclimbingmytree.com

If there is another reader who wants to share their before and after pictures as a result of reading this story I will happily post them there as well. There is also a Facebook site where you can share images and stories. Encouragement comes free!

So here are my 25 top tips to happy and healthy weight loss:

1. **Write down the top 3 reasons you want to lose weight. These will help you through the tough days.**

2. **Have a clear picture of what you want to look like, or if that is too hard, what activities you want to be able to achieve after you getter thinner and fitter.**

3. **Identify the areas of your life that are risks you need to manage actively. Travel, birthdays, work, clubs, friends? Write down how you might get through each situation and stay on track.**

4. **Download an App. that will tell you the calories you are eating and give yourself**

a target for what is ideal for your long term weight goals. Include drinks in your totals. If you want high calorie drinks you will be eating less!

5.   Make sure you have digital scales and weigh yourself to know how much you weigh right now. Ideally measure you neck or bust (I assume as a man or a woman you can work out which is best for you!) hips and waist. Remember, if the scales stay still you are probably reducing in size. Yet more encouragement.

6.   Calculate your Body Mass Index and write down how much weight you have to lose.

7.   Take some pictures of yourself when you are at your heaviest. When you have lost some weight you will be encouraged that you are smaller and this should make you even more determined not to go back!

8.   Try not to eat after 9pm. The body will be more effective at keeping you healthy if you stick to this rule.

9.   Eat a healthy breakfast of at least 15% of your total daily calorie intake to raise your metabolism and get it working well.

10. Rejoice every single day that you are in control of what you will eat. No other person can affect what YOU choose to do.

11. Weigh as much of your food as you possibly can, both at home and out of the home, to ensure you consume the correct amount rather than what you think is the correct amount!

12. Understand, you want to lose weight and keep it off, so every method you use has to be sustainable long term.

13. Tell your friends and family what you are doing and ask them to help you by not putting temptation in your way. They will, I hope, be delighted to help and encourage you.

14. Remember, if you have a bad day it is just one day and it is gone. Today is the only day you can lose any weight, not yesterday or tomorrow. It is all about right now!

15. Set milestones and celebrate each and every success. You truly are worth it.

16. Try at least one new healthy food a week to see if it is as bad as you have told yourself. Remember I discovered melon when I thought I hated it!

17. Other than trying new foods only eat food you enjoy. When you are eating right you do not want to be wasting precious calories on food you dislike.

18. Exercise is not a swear word! Find a gym that is inhabited by normal people like me and you, which operates like a whole family and where there are young and old, small and not so small, all working together to be healthy.

19. Buy a pedometer to measure your steps. Try to increase your daily count to 10,000 steps a day. Park the car a little further from work, or go for a walk. Do anything but just keep moving.

20. If at all possible, throw out any clothes that are too big for you. You will not be in need of them again and there is no way back. If you can, keep clothes that fit you and your current size, it will encourage you to keep on track.

21. Never let your weight go up by more than TWO pounds from your target. If it does rise a little more, have a very well behaved day the next day and the weight will fall off again in a day or two.

22. Eat when you are hungry and never starve yourself. Learn to eat when your body tells you it needs food.

23. Use smaller plates, smaller utensils and other tips to make food last longer and visually look like a full plate.

24. Ignore your mother, and only eat what you need to feel politely full. Please do NOT feel you have to clear your plate because that would be giving control of your weight to someone else.

25. Be intentional in all matters relating to food. Plan your intake for the day, try not to graze but take a plate of food and eat only that. Focus on what you eat and enjoy it.

Read this list at the beginning of every single week. I say to read this not because I want you to digest my words but to remind you why you are working at this and what you need to do to succeed.

I genuinely believe if you follow the advice and behaviours I have described in this book, you can be in control of your weight once and for all. Each of us has a different story and we all have inner fears. Every single person who has walked this wonderful planet has had personal battles to fight. Mine was size, and the fear that I would not ever be able to truly enjoy life with my family.

That was my main motivation and the day at Center Parcs when I once again walked into the forest with Lisa, Laura and Josh, buckled on all the safety equipment and found myself being hauled heavenwards into the treetops was one of the best days of my life. Did I care about the tree? Of course not, what I cared about was the small matter that we overwrote the memories that did not include me, and once again we were all playing together, just like we wanted! Please do not be afraid. You will succeed if you are honest with yourself and simply answer this last question...

WHAT DO YOU REALLY WANT?

NOW...GO CLIMB YOUR TREE!

Appendix 1

» Sample Menus and Meals

The following is a list of menu suggestions and calories per portion. During the weight loss period Lisa was eating approximately 1,600 calories per day and I consumed around 2,000 calories. We now choose to eat 1,800 and 2,600 Kcal per day and easily maintain our weight. The 200 Kcal we leave under the recommended daily allowances are just an insurance to make sure we do not eat too much and to account for the fact that our drinks usually contain more milk than we anticipate.

NOTES

BREAKFAST OPTIONS

50g Kellogg's All Bran (167Kcal)
120ml Skimmed Milk (41Kcal)
Low Fat Activia Yoghurt (60Kcal)
22g Quaker Granola (86Kcal)
12 Blueberries (12Kcal)
1 slice 'Crusts Away' Bread (49Kcal)
5g Low Fat spread (16Kcal)
10g Marmalade/jam (35Kcal)

TOTAL = 466Kcal

40g Kellogg's Bran Flakes (132Kcal)
120ml Semi- Skimmed Milk (59Kcal)
2 Belvita Muesli Breakfast Biscuits (114Kcal)
Muller Light Yoghurt (90Kcal)
10g Kellogg's Rice Krispies (39Kcal)

TOTAL = 434Kcal

2 Rashers Smoked Back Bacon (fat trimmed) (100Kcal)
1 Poached Egg (90Kcal)
100g Baked Beans (90Kcal)
Low Fat Activia Yoghurt (60Kcal)
1 Slice Granary Bread/Toast (100Kcal)
5g Low Fat Spread (16Kcal)

TOTAL = 456Kcal

2 Weetabix (134Kcal)
120ml Skimmed Milk (41Kcal)
Medium Banana (120Kcal)
1 McVities Waffle (118Kcal)
10ml Golden Syrup (32Kcal)

TOTAL = 445Kcal

Breakfast

NOTES

SNACK OPTIONS

25g Pretzels (95Kcal)

2 Go Ahead Yoghurt Break Biscuits (140Kcal)

Curly Wurly (115Kcal)

Mini Babybel Light (45Kcal)

15g Mini Cheddars (78Kcal)

10g Peanuts (60Kcal)

Strawberry Split Ice Cream (57Kcal)

2- Finger Kit Kat (107Kcal)

Walls Solero (90Kcal)

10g Chocolate (60Kcal)

18g Maltesers (97Kcal)

Snacks

NOTES

LUNCH OPTIONS

Pitta Bread (160Kcal)
35g Pork Loin Slices/Ham (50Kcal)
Lettuce, Cucumber, Tomato (15Kcal)
1 Packet Baked Crisps (95Kcal)
Low Fat Activia Yoghurt (60Kcal)
100g Pineapple (50Kcal)
28g Slice of Malt Loaf (88Kcal)

TOTAL = 518Kcal

Large Salad – Lettuce, Cucumber, Tomato, Celery,
20g Sweetcorn, Red Pepper (40Kcal)
100g Fresh Mussels or Prawns (90Kcal)
Slice Granary Bread (100Kcal)
5g Low Fat Spread (16Kcal)
25g Pretzels (95Kcal)
Rice Krispie Squares Bar (150Kcal)
Nectarine (60Kcal)

TOTAL = 535Kcal

Supermarket Mixed Sushi (medium) (180Kcal)
300g Fruit Salad (135Kcal)
3 Jaffa Cakes (139Kcal)

TOTAL = 454Kcal

Tesco Light Choice Lentil Soup (180Kcal)
1 slice 'Crusts Away' Bread (49Kcal)
Mr. Kipling Angel Slice (149Kcal)
Satsuma (40Kcal)
Apple (70Kcal)

TOTAL = 488Kcal

Lunch

NOTES

DINNER OPTIONS

100g Chicken (165Kcal)
250g Mixed Stir Fry Vegetables (60Kcal)
60g Sweet and Sour Sauce (69Kcal)
Nest of Noodles (178Kcal)
50g Pineapple (24Kcal)
TOTAL = 496Kcal

100g Chicken Marinated in Moroccan Spices (165Kcal)
Pitta Bread (160Kcal)
100g Potato Wedges (187Kcal)
Mixed Salad (40Kcal)
10ml Low Fat Mayonnaise (33Kcal)
TOTAL = 593Kcal

100g King Prawns (100Kcal)
150g Tesco Light Korma Sauce (120Kcal)
Mini Naan Bread (131Kcal)
Poppadum (57Kcal)
20g Mango Chutney (49Kcal)
55g white rice (raw) (200Kcal)
TOTAL = 657Kcal

75g Dried Pasta (272Kcal)
Sauce made from:
50g Tinned Tuna (58Kcal)
135g Tinned Tomatoes (23Kcal)
50g Sweetcorn (32Kcal)
¼ Red Pepper (6Kcal)
70g Mushrooms (15Kcal)
30g Courgettes (5Kcal)
20g Tomato Puree (19Kcal)
5g Parmesan Cheese (22Kcal)
TOTAL = 452Kcal

Dinner

NOTES

100g extra lean mince (125Kcal)
135g tinned tomatoes (23Kcal)
20g tomato puree
½ tbsp. gravy powder (11Kcal)
Mixed Herbs
75g dried pasta (272Kcal)
TOTAL = 449Kcal

2 Low Fat Sausages, 100g Cooked Chicken or 100g Cooked
Turkey (165Kcal)
100g Potatoes (Roasted in 1Kcal spray oil) (94Kcal)
Carrot (25Kcal)
Cabbage (20Kcal)
70g Sweetcorn (44Kcal)
50g Green beans (13Kcal)
½ tbsp. Gravy Powder (11Kcal)
Yorkshire Pudding (120Kcal)
TOTAL = 519Kcal

Small tuna steak (107Kcal)
55g white rice (raw) (200kCal)
20g Bisto White Sauce mix (99Kcal)
Carrot (25Kcal)
50g mange tout (17Kcal)
Brocoli (30Kcal)
70g mushrooms (15Kcal)
TOTAL = 493Kcal

Stuffed Mushrooms:
2 Large Flat Mushrooms (25Kcal)
40g Philadelphia Extra Light (45Kcal)
15g Low Fat Greek Yoghurt (8Kcal)
30g Bacon (71Kcal)
Slice of Gouda/Edam cheese (78Kcal
100g McCain Home Fries (181Kcal)
50g Peas (41Kcal)
50g Sweetcorn (32Kcal)
TOTAL=477Kcal

Dinner continued...

NOTES

PUDDINGS (YES YOU CAN HAVE THEM!)

60g Wall's Carte d'Or Ice Cream (82Kcal)

Cadbury's Light Chocolate Trifle (127Kcal)

Ambrosia Low Fat Rice Pudding 110g (100Kcal)

300g fruit salad (133Kcal)

50g low fat Greek yoghurt (40Kcal)

150g cooking apple (57Kcal)

Sugar-Free Angel Delight Serving (89Kcal)

60g Wall's Light Ice Cream (84Kcal)

Ambrosia Crumble pot (186Kcal)

Meringue Nest (55Kcal)

50ml Elmlea Double Light (115Kcal)

200g strawberries (64Kcal)

Mini Magnum Ice Cream (185Kcal)

Muller Rice (210Kcal)

Puddings

If you choose to follow the Very Low Calorie protocol that I used whilst taking the LDD drops then these are examples of a typical day's (*500 calories*) meals:

BREAKFAST
Mug of Black Coffee

LUNCH
Lettuce
Tomato
Cucumber
Red pepper
Beetroot
Celery
Bean Sprouts
100g Tuna

Homemade Chicken Soup:
100g Chicken per Portion
Broth from Chicken Carcass and any Vegetables

Lettuce
Tomato
Cucumber
100g Cooked Turkey
Poached Egg

DINNER
Beef Chili:
100g Extra Lean Mince
80g Tinned Tomatoes
5g Tomato Ketchup
Chili Powder to taste
Salt & Pepper
Serve on a bed of Raw Spinach

100g Chicken, Turkey, Tuna, Smoked Haddock, Lean Beef
Plus any three from:
Cabbage
Carrots
Mushrooms
Broccoli
Green Beans
Spinach
Swede

100g King Prawns
Mixed Stir Fry Vegetables
Sweet and Sour Sauce:
100ml Pineapple Juice
1 tsp. Cornflour
1 tsp. Soy Sauce
2 tsp. Brown Sugar
3 tsp. Tomato Ketchup
1 tsp. Ginger

SNACKS
Satsuma
8 Medium Strawberries
Medium Apple

It is tough but it can be done and I know several who can testify to that fact!

Very Low Cal

Appendix 2

» USEFUL LINKS
For ease of reference here are some of the sites, and resources I have used during my journey.

You can get to links to all the named suppliers following information at:
www.intentionalgroup.co.uk

If you need any other help or advice you can email *admin@intentionalgroup.co.uk*

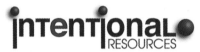

Throughout the history of mankind, the vast majority of our major achievements have been as the result of dreams and intentional plans to make those dreams reality.

- Martin Luther King dreamed of an equitable world. Yet a dream it would have remained unless he had acted upon that vision.
- Man walked on the Moon as a result of a dream and a plan of action by committed scientists in the USA.
- Numerous illnesses now have cures as a result of deliberate and focused research aimed at making the world a healthier place.
- Even in the field of sport…
- The GB Team won more medals than ever before at the London 2012 Olympic and Paralympic Games, thanks to an inspirational 8-year investment plan.
- Team Sky had a 5-year plan of action to win cycling's Tour de France, with an English rider!
- The world of Baseball revolutionised by a dream to devise a new measurement for players and performance.
- In every sphere of life people achieve amazing feats every single day in a most intentional way. Intentional Resources is a company committed to helping organisations and individuals alike to deliver the power of "intentional", to exceed their own expectations and succeed in the challenges that both life and business throw at them. Through an innovative range of books, workshops and other resources, we will simply become a helping hand for you, in whatever capacity you need to make the unbelievable believable!